618.2   Obenchain, Theodore G.
OBE   Genius belabored

WITHDRAWN
Fairhope Public Library

D0082790

SEP 0 6 2016

Genius Belabored

618.2
OBE

Genius Belabored

Childbed Fever and the Tragic Life of Ignaz Semmelweis

THEODORE G. OBENCHAIN

FAIRHOPE PUBLIC LIBRARY
501 FAIRHOPE AVE.
FAIRHOPE, AL 36532

1319548

THE UNIVERSITY OF ALABAMA PRESS
Tuscaloosa

The University of Alabama Press
Tuscaloosa, Alabama 35487–0380
uapress.ua.edu

Copyright © 2016 by the University of Alabama Press
All rights reserved.

Inquiries about reproducing material from this work should be addressed
to the University of Alabama Press.

Typeface: Trump Mediaeval

Manufactured in the United States of America
Cover photograph: Ignaz Semmelweis, age forty,
as he began writing *The Etiology, Concept, and Prophylaxis of
Childbed Fever*
Cover design: Mary-Frances Burt / Burt&Burt

∞

The paper on which this book is printed meets the minimum require-
ments of American National Standard for Information Sciences—
Permanence of Paper for Printed Library Materials, ANSI Z39.48–1984.

Library of Congress Cataloging-in-Publication Data

Names: Obenchain, Theodore G.
Title: Genius belabored : childbed fever and the tragic life of Ignaz
Semmelweis / Theodore G. Obenchain.
Other titles: Childbed fever and the tragic life of Ignaz Semmelweis
Description: Tuscaloosa : The University of Alabama Press, [2016] |
Includes bibliographical references and index.
Identifiers: LCCN 2016004130| ISBN 9780817319298 (cloth : alk.
paper) | ISBN 9780817390457 (e book)
Subjects: LCSH: Semmelweis, Ignác Fülöp, 1818–1865. |
Obstetricians—Hungary—Biography. | New mothers—Health and
hygiene—History—19th century. | Puerperal septicemia—Preven-
tion—History—19th century. | Obstetrics—History. | Hand washing.
| Sanitation.
Classification: LCC RG510.S4 O24 2016 | DDC 618.20092—dc23
LC record available at http://lccn.loc.gov/2016004130

There is a dark chapter in the history of midwifery, and it is headed—Semmelweis: left Vienna angry, returned mad.
— from Victor Robinson's
"Disraeli's Quarrels
with Authors, Semmelweis"

Contents

Figures

Genius Belabored

Introduction

In 1822, twenty-five years before Louis Pasteur announced the germ theory, Dr. William Campbell of Edinburgh, an outspoken opponent of the theory of contagion, wrote a treatise on childbed (puerperal) fever. In it he described an October 1821 event in which he had assisted in the autopsy of a young woman who had died of puerperal fever after an abortion. In preparation for a student demonstration the pelvic organs were removed, and: "I carried them in my pocket to the classroom. The same evening, without changing my clothes, I attended the delivery of a poor woman in the Cannongate; she died; next morning, I went, in the same clothes, to assist some of my pupils who were engaged with a woman . . . whom I delivered with forceps; she died; and of many others, who were seized with the disease, within a few weeks, three others shared the same fate in succession."[1]

Subsequent to those fateful few days Campbell became familiar with similar scenarios experienced by other midwives, and he was wise enough to reevaluate his anti-contagionist views. Since he still attended women in labor, he began, in 1829, to scrupulously avoid attending post-mortem examinations. Instead, he left it "to gentlemen who were not likely to be engaged with women in child-bed."[2] Such was the level of ignorance concerning disease contagion, not only within the British medical community, but with physicians throughout the Western world. Although it required eight years for Campbell to see the light, he had, at least, learned from his sad experiences and was willing to alter his behavior. Such was generally not the case. But then, in the 1840s, Ignaz Semmelweis, a man destined to function as an oracle, appeared, setting in motion all of the tensions engendered by a confrontation of enlightenment with complacent ignorance.

The tragic life of Ignaz Semmelweis could be considered a case of Cassandra syndrome, a modern version of a mythic narrative concerning an ancient Greek heroine, Cassandra, princess of Troy. When the god Apollo met Cassandra, he was so taken with her beauty that he immediately fell in love with her. Hoping to ingratiate himself to the princess, the smitten Apollo bestowed upon her the power to foretell future events. But then, as the amorous Apollo moved in, hoping to capitalize on his generosity, Cassandra spurned him. Infuriated, Apollo reciprocated in as evil a manner as he could conceive. He preserved Cassandra's ability to foresee future events, while cursing her with the quality of incredulity. She was still able to foretell the future, but she had lost the power to convince her subjects to believe her predictions. Unable to withstand the psychic tensions created between her ability to foretell future events while being disbelieved by those she aimed to protect, Cassandra was tragically driven insane. The psychodynamics of Semmelweis's fate can be viewed in a manner similar to Cassandra's. He, too, gave repeated warnings to his contemporaries concerning the contagiousness of puerperal fever, but, like Cassandra, he was preaching to an audience unable or unwilling to believe his warnings—as the disease continued to decimate masses of young women.

It seems incredible that so many seemingly intelligent people of medicine could have been so grievously wrong for so many decades. The scientific revolution, spurred by the likes of Francis Bacon, had not only begun over one hundred years before, it had even ended around the beginning of the nineteenth century. One would think that a discipline like medicine would have been sufficiently steeped in the scientific method by that time that the seeds of any promising new idea would have fallen onto fertile ground. By the 1840s, the supposed level of scientific enlightenment should have posed no problem to the acceptance of a revolutionary way of thinking about disease. But while scientific progress had occurred in some fields, such as physics and chemistry, progress remained fragmented, stratified by discipline. While certain individuals, such as Isaac Newton in mathematics and physics; Antoine Lavoisier in chemistry; Charles Lyell in geology; and others, elevated their respective fields with their illuminating work, the field of medicine lagged behind. With the sole exception of William Harvey and his elucidation of the human circulation in 1628, medicine otherwise languished in medievalism.

When asked why so little medical history is published in the modern day, noted physician and writer Lewis Thomas attributed it to the fact that the behavior of the characters in the narrative is so "pathetically bad."[3] The story of childbed fever illustrates his point. Semmelweis's saga demonstrates that when a given group, and physicians are no exception, learns some set of facts, those facts too often become immutably ingrained in the minds of that group. Then, tragically, when a valid revolutionary scientific discovery comes along, that group is either unable or unwilling to accept it. For that reason, at least until late into the nineteenth century, the process of attrition served to elevate the level of scientific consciousness more demonstrably than did the art of persuasion. As celebrated German physicist Max Planck observed, "A scientific truth does not triumph by converting its opponents and making them see the light, but rather because its opponents eventually die and a new generation grows up that is familiar with it."[4]

Semmelweis may have been surrounded by a group of intelligent men working diligently, but they labored with their blinders on. They were too complacent or too stubborn to even consider a new way of thinking. The few men of that era, such as Oliver Wendell Holmes and Semmelweis, who did struggle to solve the riddle of puerperal fever faced not only disparagement, but also overt hostility from their agnostic contemporaries. Some were driven out of town, while others faced withering criticism in the medical journals of the era. At a time when some physicians were beginning to employ scientific principles in pursuit of deadly diseases, a serious imbalance still existed between them and the medical community at large, the men to whom they preached. Too often it was scientific idealism versus slothful complacence.

Although Semmelweis died before the medical community accepted his prescient work, depriving him of the pleasure of assuming his rightful place among the giants of scientific medicine, he did finally gain recognition posthumously. Then in 2003, the late

Sherwin Nuland, medical historian and Semmelweis scholar, rendered in the Great Discoveries Series a critical and, in my opinion, unfair and unreasonable assessment of Semmelweis. In essence, he dismissed Semmelweis's role in the establishment of wound antisepsis, while ignoring his revolutionary views on disease causation. Nuland, at the least, implied that Semmelweis's career had been of marginal consequence. As a longtime casual follower of Semmelweis, I was both surprised and intrigued enough by Nuland's criticisms to study the subject in more depth with thoughts of setting the record straight—as I saw it. Further research, however, revealed insights as to why Semmelweis acted the way he did, insights that, as a consequence, render Nuland's criticisms less relevant. For decades medical historians have recognized that Semmelweis's tortured life was dominated by some type of unidentifiable mental ailment. They have, as well, debated over his autopsy findings, considering such diagnoses as neurosyphilis, Alzheimer's disease, or some other less specific degenerative condition of the brain. In the latter part of the book, I offer a diagnosis that not only best explains his living eccentricities but also ties in well with the abnormalities discovered in his brain at autopsy.

But without even considering the intriguing points above, this story stands alone, a tragically stirring narrative of a man with flagrant in-born flaws, working against impossible odds, who devoted his life to the solution of a great scourge that had been decimating the feminine half of the populace for more than a century. Semmelweis solved the mystery of contagion while struggling "rudderless" in the murky waters of clinical obstetrics, relying purely on empirical observations decades before the advent of the germ theory.

Finally, for reader clarity, some unusual but easily understood medical terms require definition. The lay term, *childbed fever*, and the medical term, *puerperal fever*, are synonymous. The word *puerperal*, which appears throughout the book, is derived from the Latin root "*puer*," meaning child. The root gives rise to: puerperal, meaning with child; "*puerperae*," meaning pregnant women; and "*puerperium*," meaning the duration of pregnancy and the few days after delivery. Another frequently used term is "*accoucheur*," the French word for obstetrician. It was used widely, not only in France, but across much of Europe. "*Parturition*" is another word used throughout, meaning to give birth. A *"parturient"* is therefore one giving birth and is synonymous with puerpera or puerperae (plural). The word *"gravid,"* from the root word *"gravis,"* meaning heavy, is an adjective, as in gravid uterus. *"Gravidae"* is plural, i.e., more than one expectant woman.

All of the facts presented in this work are true. However, in the first chapter, the characters, with the exception of Semmelweis, have been fictionalized to better illustrate the factual picture of puerperal fever as it confronted the obstetricians of the 1840s. With that brief introduction, the path to the tragic life of Semmelweis is set.

Puerperal Fever

On a sweltering midnight in July 1846, Erna, obstetrical head nurse at the gigantic Vienna General Hospital (Allegemeine Krankenhaus) approached the entrance to the physician's on-call room. Looking up at the door, she gave a series of crisp, rapid knocks, only to have the urgency of her visit entirely wasted on the room's occupant, Ignaz Semmelweis, newly appointed assistant accoucheur (obstetrician) in the Obstetrics Department's First Division. He lay in his call quarters in the deep sleep of exhaustion, having just endured a hectic twenty-four hour marathon of deliveries, a rude introduction to his first week on duty. Finally aroused from sleep, he staggered to open the door, leaning heavily upon its casing. Upon seeing Semmelweis, Erna began expressing her unease concerning a young mother who appeared to be developing medical problems a mere twenty-four hours after her delivery. Realizing that the seriousness of this problem would require his visiting the ward, Semmelweis turned to a washbowl, throwing some cool water onto his face, giving Erna just enough time for a quick visual assessment of his quarters. Furnished with only a chair, a chest of drawers, and a straw-stuffed mattress lying upon something more like a cot than a bed, it was depressingly Spartan by any definition. For a man only two years out of medical school, being the obstetrical assistant was a position equivalent to a modern chief-resident in a major university teaching hospital. Any physician successfully surviving the rigors of his chosen specialty at this famous Vienna hospital could be virtually assured of a prestigious position somewhere in Europe upon leaving the confines of arguably the finest hospital on the continent.

Semmelweis, by now, had become fully aware of his surroundings. After donning a cover gown, giving his moistened hair an obligatory swipe with the palms of his hands, he exited his room, proceeding with Erna along a corridor poorly illuminated by lantern-light. After traversing two lying-in wards of expectant women, he entered a cavernous gymnasium-like room with beds arranged in rows, one along each wall and a third coursing down the center. So closely arranged were the adjacent beds that each occupant could easily reach out, both right and left, and touch the outstretched arm of her neighbor. Lack of personal space on such wards was a given. If one wished for privacy, the best she could hope for was some empathetic nurse placing curtains around her bed. As Semmelweis approached the proper row of beds, peering through the lantern light, he immediately recognized his patient, a puerile-appearing sixteen year old, lying supine, with eyes closed. He could not escape the irony; she seemed a mere child on Monday, yet was a mother on Tuesday. Just to be certain he had the right patient, he made that confirmatory glance at the chalkboard above her bed displaying the name, "Renate." She had been a resident of the ward for the past six weeks, that is, since the time her pregnancy made it impossible to continue work as a chambermaid for a prominent Viennese family. Renate, like most of her ward-mates, was going through the delivery without the support of the child's father. After she informed him of her gravid state, he pulled a sudden disappearing act, leaving her alone to grapple with her sudden change of fortune. Still, she had actually looked forward to the birth of her child, unlike many of the single women on the ward, despite the expected financial hardship brought on by single parenthood. She enjoyed the good fortune of having a sister and some devoted friends who had volunteered to help with her child-care.

Renate's delivery had presented a problem for Semmelweis and his team. Her labor had progressed slowly and inefficiently, something not uncommon in primiparous women, those experiencing their first deliveries. With his usual retinue of four medical students in tow, Semmelweis had closely monitored her progress through labor with frequent pelvic examinations. Each student, by ministerial edict, was obliged to examine the patient after Semmelweis. What better way for a student to become familiar with the changing dynamics of labor? Ordinarily, a solo accoucheur might carry out three to four exams during the eighteen hours of such a difficult labor. But, taking the four medical students and their examinations into consideration, in reality, four exams meant twenty individual internal probings over the full course of labor. Yet, one could argue that being vigilant was wise. Serial examinations enabled the obstetrician to remain alert to upcoming problems. He could intervene more expeditiously should some emergency arise. One could better assess how the uterus was progressing through labor either by direct palpation of the abdomen, or by feeling with the finger tip. Were the contractions strong? Was the cervix dilating and effacing (thinning out) adequately? Was the proper part of the fetus engaging appropriately in the upper pelvis before beginning its descent into the lower part of the birth canal? The earlier the obstetrician detected some problem with the fetus or labor, the more timely could his intervention be on behalf of both mother and fetus. If a child presented in a mal-rotated state, with perhaps an arm and shoulder engaging the pelvic brim, a simple manual rotation of the fetus by an alert obstetrician could avert disaster, saving the life of both mother and child. Certain other problems might require the rare employment of forceps or even, as a last resort, a Caesarean section.

Although Renate's labor had been difficult and prolonged, she required none of these measures, finally delivering spontaneously after eighteen painfully long hours. Both mother and son appeared to have survived the ordeal with no obvious problem. Per hospital protocol, Renate walked back to her bed, unassisted, three hours after delivery. With liberal doses of laudanum (tincture of opium) she could finally relax. Now, nearly twenty hours later, as Semmelweis examined her in the flickering lantern light, he could feel the dried residue of sweat on her face and in her hair. Noticing her parched lips and dry tongue, he recalled having admonished her, shortly after delivery, to begin drinking the barley water at her bedside as he exited the ward around 4:00 AM. Now, with her vomiting, fluid intake posed a problem.

Even though her pulse was only mildly elevated, barely over one hundred beats per minute, it was too high for this stage of her delivery. The nurse reported a temperature of 100° F, now twenty hours after delivery. She appeared moderately distressed, complaining of nausea, malaise, and some ill-defined abdominal pain centered just above her pubic bone, but she was alert and capable of full activity. As he applied a stethoscope to her abdomen, only the rarest of bowel sounds were evident, indicating a worrisome lack of bowel function. Semmelweis had his suspicions about the dreaded puerperal fever, but in her present condition he could detect no definitive signs that would make the diagnosis a certainty. Nor could he be absolutely certain of her future course at such an early point in time. Such uncertainty allowed him to put up a positive front to the patient without feeling dishonest. He informed Renate that he suspected an inflammation in her uterus (metritis) or fallopian tubes (salpingitis). As long as the inflammation remained localized, it might very well resolve of its own accord. He offered a treatment plan to her: more laudanum for her pain and the application of abdominal poultices. In spite of her nausea, the nursing staff would continue encouraging fluids, the barley water, to minimize her dehydration.

Now that Semmelweis was fully awake, his sleep interrupted, he remained up, retreating to another part of the ward to address other miscellaneous items. When he returned to Renate an hour later for an update on her symptoms, even from a distance he noted a worrisome subtle change. While lying on her back, she subconsciously held both hips and knees in a flexed attitude. Something about that position brought her relief—a reduction in a painful tension she sensed emanating from her lower belly. Alerted, Semmelweis pressed his fingers into her lower abdominal wall, causing her some nondescript discomfort. More significantly, when he suddenly released his pressure, her pain increased dramatically, to the point of making her cry out. She had rebound pain, an early sign of peritonitis, a serious inflammation of her abdominal lining.

Despite being a comparative novice, Semmelweis had already witnessed too many heartrending cases of puerperal fever beginning in just this manner. He had an ominous foreboding—a dread for what was likely in store for this innocent young woman—and sensed the incipient stages of a nightmarish scenario. It reduced Semmelweis, this idealistic caregiver, used to being in control, to the uncomfortable position of observer, powerless to slow the fulminating process in any definitive manner.

Semmelweis made brief visits, short spot-checks, to her bedside throughout the night. By 2:00 AM her pulse remained elevated, while her temperature had risen to 102°F. Her abdominal pain was worse. Although she could respond appropriately to most questions, she had become delirious, tremulous, and confused. On this exam, Semmelweis noted red streaks, central lines sprouting off short tributaries at random, like scarlet sprigs of thyme, coursing from her upper-inner thighs along the pale-white skin of her lower abdominal wall. Adding to his disquiet, he discovered small, swollen, bluish-black spots of discoloration in the skin of her private parts. Of equal concern, her lochia, the normal discharge after delivery, had become strongly malodorous. It was the stench of putrefaction. As he stood over her supine figure, Semmelweis noted the sudden onset of uncontrollable shaking throughout her body, accompanied by a chattering of teeth that persisted for several minutes. To the uninitiated, her movements might have been mistaken for a convulsion. But Semmelweis recognized the event for what it was, the onset of blood "crasis," a mysterious, fermentive degeneration taking place within her bloodstream—a grave and irreversible development. Too bad his medical students were home in bed, sleeping through such a teachable moment. The full understanding of blood crasis, or "blood poisoning" as an infection within the bloodstream was not yet appreciated. In fact, it would take decades and full elucidation of the germ theory before physicians recognized the shaking and chattering for what it truly represented—the sudden invasion of massive numbers of bacteria into the bloodstream. But Semmelweis, through prior cases, was experienced enough to know that Renate's future was now all too clear. Her uncontrollable rigors signaled the onset of fulminating disease, her calamitous descent over the medical precipice. In this era before antibiotics, her death was a foregone conclusion.

After a short and fitful night, Semmelweis arose around 6:00 AM. Per his usual routine, he proceeded immediately to the dead house, the hospital morgue, a converted old rifle factory where autopsies were performed on all patients dying within the hospital. Semmelweis had been fortunate to work out an agreement with his pathology professor that allowed him to perform autopsies on all patients dying within the maternity department. Puerperal fever represented, by far, the largest percentage of such deaths. After completing his morning dissections over the course of several hours, he gave a perfunctory wipe of his hands and arms with a dry cloth. Next he washed them thoroughly with soap and water. Still, as he left the morgue, negotiating the stairway to the obstetrics floor, he could not help but notice. Not that it was anything out of the ordinary, but his hands still reeked of putrefaction, the fetid odor of death. But he was used to that. Despite the most vigorous scrubbing with soap and water the aroma was not easily washed away. After performing autopsies daily over a period of time one became inured to the odor. It seemed to penetrate all layers of the skin. By the time he reached the maternity ward, all thoughts of putrefaction had been pushed to the back of his mind. His concerns switched, instead, to the patients awaiting his attention.

As he approached Renate's bed, Semmelweis was hardly surprised to see that she was worse. Obviously, the feeble attempts at treatment had been pitifully inadequate. The nurse reported a fever of 104° with a pulse of 150. Bending closer to her, he noted that her lips and nail beds were a dusky-blue. When he addressed her by name she mumbled something about Hans, the absentee father of her newborn, but her ramblings were largely unintelligible. To better assess her level of consciousness, Semmelweis rubbed a knuckle across her breast bone causing her eyes to open briefly. She raised her arms moving them about in an aimless manner. By now, her abdomen was rigid, like the skin of a drum, and so distended it could be detected from across the ward. As paroxysms of pressure coursed through her abdomen she shrieked out in pain. Those red streaks, incipient when he had first seen her abdomen at midnight, had now coalesced into full bloom. The massively swollen soft tissues of her private area had turned a shade of deep blue-black. Deprived of their blood supply, these tissues were dying. Then, as Semmelweis stood at her bedside, Renate suffered a true convulsion, beginning first with a twitching of her face, then her arm and leg, all confined to her right side. Within seconds the seizure spread to all of her extremities, continuing for nearly a minute. Then a slow decrescendo of spasms ensued until she lay completely immobile, utterly flaccid throughout, not even breathing for nearly a full minute. Just as the nurses began wondering if she were dead, her breathing returned in a slow crescendo, along with improvement in her coloring. But she was moribund, flaccid, and deeply unconscious. It was all but over.

Charged with other patient responsibilities, Semmelweis and his medical students continued on with their working rounds. Still, as he progressed from one bed to another, he could not help but cast nervous glances back to where Renate lay. Finally, when he observed the nurses pulling the duvet over her face he knew it was over. Her body would remain in bed and on the ward for hours until hospital staff could make a place for her in the morgue. She would be on Semmelweis's autopsy schedule for the following day—another in a long line of tragic deaths. One could not help but reflect on the sad ending for this young woman who had entered the hospital in such a cheerful and optimistic state. She was now but another in a long line of new mothers succumbing to puerperal fever, the scourge of maternity wards the world over. One wry observation circulating around the morgue from time to time highlighted an all too frequent grim scenario: "Enter the hospital, have an operation, end up on the dissecting slab," or, expressed more tersely, "Diagnose, Operate, Die, Dissect." High mortality rates from puerperal fever had been a problem for over one hundred years, persisting well into the nineteenth century. As late as 1879, noted French accoucheur, Jacques Hervieux, observed, "Epidemic puerperal fever is to women what war is to men. Like war, it cuts down the healthiest, bravest, and most essential part of the population; like war, its victims are in the prime of their lives."[1]

Even though Semmelweis brought a high level of enthusiasm to his dissections in the early stages, the continual onslaught of puerperal fever victims gave him no opportunity to gain any emotional respite from dealing with the deaths of young women in his charge. Entering the morgue each morning preparing for his string of autopsies did little to assuage his angst. Handling such events had posed little problem for him when he was a medical student, merely passing through the morgue and a course in obstetrics. Objectifying the dead and dying had been easier. While that stark image of some anonymous, hoary human form lying supine on the autopsy table may have made an impression on him, he was not personally connected to it. Any image of the unknown dead that may have occupied his mind immediately slipped out of mind as he left the premises, going on to other pursuits.

But now, as prime caregiver to these young women, the situation was far different. His close identification with them was inescapable. However brief the interaction with his young patients might have been in their days of confinement, he knew them. In Renate's case, they had shared some light moments. She had even related how eagerly she anticipated her child's birth. How could he not vividly recall Renate's personality? Seeing her body lying supine on the autopsy slab, one would have to be heartless to blithely dissociate from her past, and from her tragic recent history. With the usual waxing and waning of puerperal fever on the wards as many as perhaps a score of women per week died under his care. He autopsied them, one and all, in an unremitting scenario. The steady drumbeat of young women dying on the wards, their bodies then arriving in the morgue week after week weighed heavily on the young assistant.

In preparation for Renate's autopsy, Semmelweis arranged the appropriate papers and paraphernalia, while the technician aligned the scalpels, saws, hooks, and rongeurs in order of easy access. In the 1840s, all autopsies and cadaver dissections were performed with bare hands. Protective gloves, an invention of William Halstead of Johns Hopkins Hospital, would not come into general use until the 1890s. After rolling his sleeves up well above his elbows, Semmelweis grabbed a scalpel. He began by sliding the knife upwards, from pubic bone to the bottom of Renate's rib cage before bifurcating the incision into its final Y-shape. As the scalpel penetrated the peritoneum, the deepest layer of abdominal tissues, an overwhelming stench of putrefaction escaped into the air, a smell so strong and pervasive that he reflexively turned away, covering his nose with flexed elbow, waiting for the smell to dissipate. Some medical students had to briefly exit the room for fear of vomiting. After recovering, Semmelweis next spread the abdominal walls laterally revealing a large volume of slimy, yellow-white fluid, termed, for lack of a better word, an "exudate." The fluid, perhaps three liters in all, had gravitated in between her abdominal organs. Some pathologists correctly recognized the exudate as pus, but to others it was considered to be a coagulum of fermented milk. In fact, the real explanation behind such fluid was unknown. During any deep dissection of internal organs such as this, it was common for the dissector's forearms, along with his shirt sleeves, to become soiled with bodily fluids up to a level around the elbows. In fact, at this point, Semmelweis had to enlist help from a passer-by to roll his unraveled sleeves, once again, back up above his elbows.

After using strips of cloth to wipe the cavity free of its milky exudate, Semmelweis next turned his attention to the peritoneal membrane, the thin lining of the inner abdominal wall. Grasping forceps in his left hand and cotton swabs in his right, he peeled a portion of the peritoneal lining away from the inner abdominal wall, much as one might skin a deer. He demonstrated to the students in attendance how the peritoneal membrane carpets not only the inner lining of bodily cavities, but all organs within the abdominal and chest cavities as well. In its normal state the peritoneal membrane is so thin and transparent that it would be nearly identical to a sheet of modern-day Saran Wrap. Semmelweis pointed out to his student charges how, in the case at hand, the inflammatory process of puerperal fever had dramatically altered the peritoneum. No longer thin and transparent, it was an opaque, yellow-white carpet of thickened tissue, slimy as the skin of a Beluga sturgeon swimming in the Danube nearby.

With the dramatic inflammatory changes in her external, private parts, seen on bedside exam, it was not surprising to encounter comparable findings inside her pelvis. The uterus and its surrounding tissues were obviously the most affected. Semmelweis had recognized long ago that those tissues around the uterus represented the epicenter of inflammation. Inflammation was so severe that it had occluded all arteries and veins in the area, depriving the surrounding tissues of their blood supply. Necrotic (dead) pelvic tissue predominated. Pockets of pus lay scattered around the pelvic floor. The uterus, fallopian tubes, and ovarian areas were uniformly encased in spider web-like strands of inflammatory adhesions, coursing to bowel and pelvic brim nearby.

As Semmelweis continued his dissection up the abdomen, he removed the liver. Slicing through it with a long knife, as one would a loaf of bread, he demonstrated to the students the minute foci of inflammatory cells, a diffuse scattering of micro-abscesses. The abscesses were small only because of the brevity of Renate's illness. The longer one's illness persisted, the greater amount of time ex-

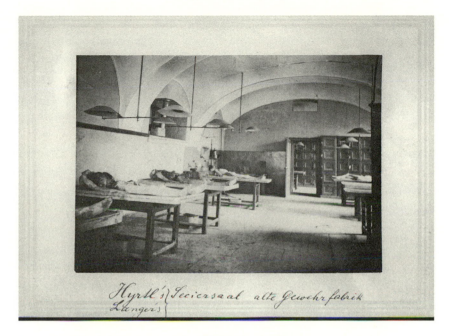

Figure 1. The morgue at Vienna General Hospital, a converted rifle factory, in 1874. Semmelweis performed his many autopsies on victims of puerperal fever here. Copper plate by Joseph and Peter Schaffer. Courtesy of Vienna University's Josephinum.

isted for the abscesses to mature and grow larger. A similar slicing through the kidneys revealed the same minute lesions, distributed at random per the vagaries of circulation. This random scattering of small abscesses, a consequence of septicemia, is referred to as a miliary process, a poetic reference to the millet seed. If one were to open an artery and inject millet seeds into the circulation he would note the same random distribution of minute seeds not only down to the capillary level but extending through it into all tissues of the body, the kidneys, the liver, the bones, and even the nervous system.

After cutting through her ribs with a rongeur, Semmelweis lifted the sternum off of Renate's body, much like lifting the lid of a trunk, hinged by tissues at the base of her neck. Gazing down on the contents within, he noted the same malodorous, milky, yellow-white fluid that he had encountered in the abdomen. After cleansing the chest of the liquid, he removed her lungs. Pus was evident in and around the larger blood vessels. To the students in attendance he once again pointed out the multiple, nascent abscesses scattered throughout the lung tissue proper, identical to the findings in other organs.

Next Semmelweis incised her heart in such a manner that all four chambers were exposed. Each valve displayed multiple vegetations, that is, collections of micro-organisms and dead tissue remnants, growing on their surfaces. Had Renate survived longer these vegetations would have matured and spread through the entirety of the valves, rendering them incompetent, unable to effectively control the forward (systolic) flow of blood, or prevent its backflow during the diastolic phase, with each beat of the heart.

Before calling Renate's postmortem exam complete Semmelweis was obligated to examine one last organ system. Her terminal convulsion and deep coma meant that her nervous system was almost certainly involved. Given its full encasement in bone, just elevating a skull cap to allow for removal of the brain was a time-consuming task. Once completed, he inspected the brain's surface. The gyri, or natural ridges, were swollen, while the sulci, or valleys, revealed linear distributions of yellow pus gravitated down into the recesses. Semmelweis detected the same random scattering of micro-abscesses throughout the brain's surface. One such abscess, in a more advanced state, had the distinct margins of a walnut shell, filled with a yellow liquid center. Lying deeper within the brain surface on the left side, it was the likely cause of her terminal right-sided convulsion.

Adding to the family tragedy, Renate's infant son had to be placed in the nearby Royal Foundling Home at the time of her death, to be wet-nursed and cared for by others. Given a happier scenario, he would have remained at her bedside, day and night, until the two left the hospital for home. Sadly, he died a day later than Renate—an all-too-common accompaniment of puerperal fever. Such infants, infected through their mother's circulation, deteriorated in a manner strikingly similar to that of their mothers. High fever, rapid pulse, mental deterioration progressing into a delirium, to coma, and finally, to death was the scenario common to them all. At autopsy, the tissues surrounding the newborn's umbilical cord remnant revealed red and black marks, that inflammatory prelude to tissue death. Internal exam of Renate's son exhibited the same changes wrought by sepsis—yellow-white exudates throughout his abdominal and chest cavities. Blood, placed in a glass tube for one hour, revealed a layer of buoyant pus cells resting on the top, like cream rising to the surface of milk. His major organs, such as the liver and lungs, contained numerous small aggregations of pus cells, nascent abscesses consequent to the dreaded blood "crasis."

How had puerperal fever become such a problem? While recognized as a disease since the time of Hippocrates, it did not pose a significant threat for hundreds of years. If one were to attribute the ascendency of puerperal fever to any single cause, either proximate or remote, it would be the Industrial Revolution. Larger cities, as the sites for new and burgeoning industries, became magnets for jobs, causing a new workforce to move *en masse* from country to city. Such a massive move of people had its consequences—overcrowding with its inevitable centralized concentration of filth, sewage, and industrial pollution. Still, scientists would not begin to understand the actual cause of individual cases of childbed fever until the mid-1870s, when they learned that concentrations of disease-causing bacteria thrived in such filthy, overcrowded, urban settings.

Before the mid-eighteenth century, maternity care, whether playing out in a municipal or rural location, had always been an in-home, feminine event, administered by midwives or amateur care-givers, women stirred into action to help a friend or family member through a difficult event. But circumstances changed around 1750, when physicians and trained midwives began assuming the dominant role in this natural biological event. Such a change in care was easy to justify on theoretical grounds. Was it not safer to have the professionally trained take charge of the process? As a consequence, the site of deliveries changed as well, moving from home to hospital. Not coincidentally, it was at this same time that the numbers of women succumbing to puerperal fever began to increase. By 1800, all major cities, such as Vienna, Berlin, Paris, and Gottingen had erected large lying-in hospitals, facilities in which young women presented themselves in ever-increasing numbers. Centralization of care seemed a laudable goal for any city— shelter from the storm in a caring environment, supplemented by good nutrition and access to skilled medical care.[2]

Physicians recognized that some connection, however nebulous, existed between contagion and puerperal fever. Toward that end, most European hospital wards were designed and built by architects and city planners as cavernous, open auditoria, fully compliant with the most widely accepted theories of contagion. Authorities were concerned about the large number of patients living within the confines of hospital walls, inhaling and exhaling filthy, miasmatic air. With no ductworks or energy sources, save for heat, they put great trust in cross-ventilation—that natural cleanser—to minimize the incidence of puerperal infection; clean air streamed in through windows on one side of the building and out of windows on the opposite side. By keeping the windows open continuously, ten feet off the floor and out of reach of the nurses, robust cross-ventilation was ensured.[3] Even in the colder winter months windows remained open. Specially insulated Meissner-jacket furnaces, often two to a large ward, blew warm air in and around the resting patients.[4]

But this valued cross-ventilation came at a high price in the form of compromised patient privacy. Wards were deliberately left open, with no partitioning, no hallways or separate rooms that might tend to diminish such ventilation around the beds. Patients lay in their assigned spots, side-by-side, each in full view of their neighbors. Beds were deliberately arranged along the length of the wards in rows beneath the windows. Another row or two of beds might be arranged down the center of the ward if patient census demanded it. Expectant and new mothers lay on straw mattresses covered with woolen blankets, while newborns remained with their mothers constantly, both night and day. Each floor contained at least one privy in a corner, but through bitter experience, hospital authorities prohibited patients from using them. After discovering that a number of young mothers had hurled their newborns into the privies and to their deaths several stories below, guardrails were built around each privy on every floor. Nurses employed bedpans for all bodily functions, in effect, giving the mothers no need to get anywhere near the privies. Proximity might breed temptation.[5]

Hospital staff did make efforts to maintain a certain level of cleanliness. In the ideal scenario, they changed bed linens daily and woolen blankets every four to eight days. Every eight days the floors were freshly scrubbed, and each patient's mattress was emptied, then restuffed with fresh, clean straw. Hospital walls received a new coat of white paint annually.[6] Not surprisingly, in the reality of day-to-day practice these ideals were not always met.

During Semmelweis's assistantship, eight obstetrical wards existed with a total capacity of two hundred beds distributed between the first and second stories. Thirty beds were reserved for those in active labor. Hospital admissions, which alternated daily between the two divisions, could vary from 50 to as many as 120 patients per day. Division I admitted four days per week, while the second division admitted the remaining three days. Overcrowding was a constant. To maintain that delicate equilibrium between patients in need and bed availability, every healthy new mother was obligated to leave the hospital by her ninth day after delivery. Adding to the functional complexities of a busy ward, the department was charged with training 150 to 200 accoucheurs and 260 to 300 midwives annually. Noon hours were reserved for the instruction of medical students in the mechanics of delivery using adult female and infant cadavers. At the same time, outside the confines of the obstetrical department, student midwives learned the same mechanics on an artificial model, a leather phantom, and fetal cadavers.[7]

At Vienna General Hospital, gravid young women typically spent the terminal two months of their pregnancy in the hospital, all care and sustenance free of charge. In exchange, these poverty-stricken women were obligated to maintain the space around their beds and to freely submit to any and all examinations by medical students and faculty. As "teaching material" such expectant women provided a valuable service to both university students and the state. By the daily observation of a woman's last two months of gestation, and the opportunity to participate in all deliveries, students were provided with an incomparable chance to learn the basics of obstetrics.

City fathers, in their planning, hoped that one other social scourge, inherently related to unwed gravid women, might be solved through centralization of care in maternity hospitals. Young mothers, typically unable to earn a living because of their maternal obligations, committed infanticide with disturbing frequency. In some large cities the problem proved so pervasive that hospitals provided sidewalk turnstiles (*Routa*), maternal "lazy Susans," whereby mothers could gain their freedom by merely inserting their swaddled charges into an enclosed receptacle. A simple half-revolution of the turnstile, 180 degrees, and hospital staff, sitting on the other side of the wall, received the infant. The entire transaction was completed silently and anonymously—no questions asked, no explanations offered.[8]

Closely affiliated with the lying-in hospitals were the so-called "foundling homes," facilities lying in close proximity, designed to care for newborns of the women who either died in childbirth or were unwilling or physically unable to care for their offspring for whatever reason. In this era, decades before any expertise or knowledge of intravenous fluid administration existed, mortality rates of 50 percent were common in such foundling homes due mainly to epidemics of puerperal fever plus rampant outbreaks of infantile dysentery.

Puerperal fever accounted for approximately half of all maternal deaths. From the mid-nineteenth century to the 1930s, the malady ranked second only to tuberculosis as a cause of death in women.[9] No wonder the feelings of frustration for the treating physician. Safest were decentralized home deliveries. Here mortality rates, whether attended by midwives or physicians, remained around 0.45 percent. Hospital epidemics, in which mortality rates might rise by as much as twenty to sixty times that figure, were typically the most hazardous.[10] Even with the best of care, physicians considered a mortality rate of 1 percent the ideal, the best achievable. To the modern mind it is difficult to understand how the public could have tolerated such abysmally high death rates. Ignorance and attitude played a big part. Many women entered the hospital oblivious to the dangers lurking there, while others just had a generally optimistic outlook. So what if 15 percent of the women died? That meant that 85 percent got through the ordeal unscathed—still fairly decent odds.

The lay term, childbed fever, synonymous with its medical counterpart, puerperal fever, evolved into common usage in the 1700s, as deaths associated with labor and delivery soared. Strange that such a natural process had become a major threat to an expectant woman. Women from even the most primitive of societies had been delivering in a safe, inherently decentralized manner for millennia. As puerperal fever became more prevalent, a spectrum of different disease manifestations emerged. For lesser forms of puerperal infections, physicians commonly named the disease for the organ most affected. If it were the uterus, it was called metritis; fallopian tubes, salpingitis, and so on. These localized, less threatening forms of disease commonly resolved spontaneously with time.

But if the infection spread out of the pelvic region into the peritoneal (abdominal) cavity, the picture of the disease and its prognosis changed radically. So dramatic was the new development of peritonitis that its presence came to define the disease. Some physicians referred to this level of infection as puerperal peritonitis, but to the majority, puerperal fever still remained the preferred name. On examination, the physician could "feel" the peritoneal inflammation—the excruciatingly painful swollen belly—tight as a drum, the rebound pain, and the absence of bowel sounds. No need for argument; full-blown peritonitis represented a grave development—it was but a short time from peritonitis until sepsis, or "degradation" of the blood, occurred. Physicians generally preferred the less specific terms, "crasis" or "dyscrasia," meaning an imbalance or degeneration of blood components. From a practical standpoint, once blood crasis developed, death was inevitable. The only question was how long before it happened?

Of course, physicians of the 1840s were completely ignorant of not only what caused puerperal fever, but even how it developed in the individual patient. While they recognized sepsis, infection in the blood, as a life-threatening condition, all were virtually ignorant of the role that bacteria played in its origin. It would be nearly two decades, until 1857, before Louis Pasteur even proposed his theory of germs to the French Academy of Medicine. So slowly did the wheels of science move that another twenty-two years would transpire before Pasteur demonstrated convincingly, in 1879, that the "string of pearls" (streptococci), seen only with the aid of a microscope, was the true causative agent of puerperal fever. Physicians did not even begin to gain competence in using the microscope in any general way until the late nineteenth century.

Physicians remained equally ignorant of another fact: the peritoneal surface is itself a highly absorptive membrane; just how absorptive they would not discover until decades later. With the development of anesthetics physicians discovered that they could sustain a patient's anesthetized state merely by injecting anesthetics directly into the peritoneal cavity. Or, one could administer fluids by the same route, almost as effectively as by the intravenous route. The peritoneum was that absorptive. In 1920, well after Semmelweis's time, scientists pioneering the technique of dialysis discovered that even waste products could be removed across the peritoneal membrane. If various compounds are able to gain entrance into the blood stream through this highly absorptive membrane, it should not be surprising that bacteria, once they have established colonies on the peritoneal surface, have similar access to the circulation. As millions of bacteria invade the bloodstream the patient experiences teeth-chattering rigors—the bedside pronouncement of sepsis. If sepsis is fully established and remains untreated, it ushers in death by inducing failure of multiple organ systems. Not until the advent of sulfa drugs in the 1930s would any definitive treatment exist for infectious diseases as a group, including childbed fever.[11]

One other peculiar variant of the disease deserves mention. In many cases of peritonitis, physicians did note, after the onset of the full-blown condition, one inexplicable and ironic happening. Patients stuck in that pre-terminal state transitioned, inexplicably, into an awake, fully oriented, peaceful quietude, no more moaning—their ailment seemingly gone. Had the peritoneum recovered in some way? The change, dramatic enough to lull a neophyte physician into a state of optimism, was, in reality, nothing more than a prelude to death. More experienced physicians postulated that, as the gangrenous tissues within the abdomen died, the nerves that mediated the pain died as well.[12] An observant young physician should only be fooled once.

Such were the characteristics of the disease confronting Semmelweis about the time that he began his career in obstetrics. Since physicians had no understanding of its cause, nor any effective means of treating puerperal fever, the disease struck terror in the hearts of patients and caregivers alike. As the renowned American professor of obstetrics, Charles Meigs, so wistfully observed in 1848, any young parturient dying of puerperal fever was a desecration: "Even small pox, which reduces the fairest form of humanity to a mass of breathing corruption, cannot be looked upon with greater awe . . . There is something so touching in the death of a woman who has recently given birth to her child; something so mournful in the disappointment of cherished hopes; something so pitiful in the disordered condition of the new-born helpless creature, forever deprived of those tender cares and caresses so necessary for it—that the hardest heart is sensible to the catastrophe."[13]

Adding to the fear and disappointment engendered by puerperal fever, once the disease became fully manifest, the physician was rendered as feckless as one standing on a river's edge watching a loved one's descent over a waterfall—a mere observer with nothing to offer but some hand wringing and sympathy. If one understood the cause of puerperal fever, perhaps the disease could at least be prevented, but such was not the case. To Semmelweis, the disease was as frightening as it was to his colleagues. Yet, unlike his colleagues, Semmelweis saw in puerperal fever a troubling dichotomy. While he was driven to a state of chronic melancholy from observing the large numbers of women dying under his care, at the same time, the disease represented his noble challenge—one that would consume the rest of his life.

Most accoucheurs of the 1840s coped with the huge numbers of dead young mothers by merely turning aside in quiet resignation. High mortality rates were just the way things were. Settling into an uneasy coexistence with such an insoluble problem was the easiest route to follow. But Semmelweis was different. Some unique, indefinable aspect of his persona drove him to reject such complacency. He would dedicate his life, in a tragically literal sense, to the conquest of this dreaded killer of young mothers.

Prodrome

Ignaz Fulop Semmelweis was born to Josef and Therezia Semmelweis on 1 July 1818, in the Taban, an older section of Buda, originally settled by Serbians in the 1700s. Buda, the mountainous section
on the western bank of the Danube, was initially a city distinct from
Pest, which lay to the east of the river. Ignaz, the fifth of ten children,
grew up in a close-knit, happy Catholic family. In spite of residing in
a poor and politically repressed country, and hailing from a family
tree with no particularly illustrious antecedents, young Ignaz would
never have to worry about finances during his younger formative
years. Josef, the father, enjoyed great success as an influential grocer.

Ignaz's numerous biographers consistently describe the young
man in his early years as bright, well-adjusted, energetic, warm of
heart, imaginative, and physically strong. One of them, William
Sinclair, referred to him as a "clever boy with a ready tongue, full
of energy, warmth of heart and imagination."[1] In fact, even into
his high school and college years, his personality seemed so felicitous, so eager to please, that it sometimes made him appear juve-
nile, years younger than his stated age. Years later, a fellow student,
Ignaz Hirschler, described him as being a happy, cheerful person,
well liked by both teachers and fellow students. He was humble
and modest, with a sort of childish, naive mindset, one who lived
the moment fully without inhibition.[2] Yet Semmelweis revealed a
hint of fragility in his own psyche years later, when he described
himself as possessing an innate distaste and aversion to any form
of controversy.[3] With such personality traits he enjoyed great popularity throughout all stages of his youth. Ignaz was stereotypically

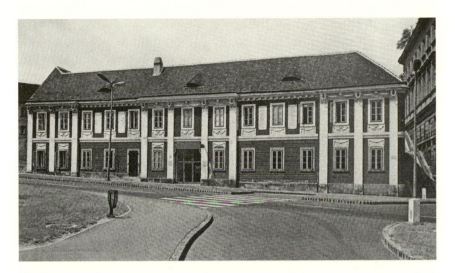

Figure 2. Ignaz Semmelweis's birth home and current site of the Semmelweis Museum in Buda on the eastern side of the Danube River. Buda Castle and military fortifications, out of view, occupy the higher ground to the right of the photo.

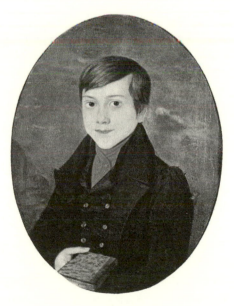

Figure 3. Oil painting of Ignaz Semmelweis in 1830, at the age of twelve, by Lénart Landau (1790–1868).

FAIRHOPE PUBLIC LIBRARY

1319548 Ingram 9-16 29.95

Teutonic in appearance, with lucid, grey-blue eyes and fine, straight blond hair. He was middling in stature and mildly corpulent. Frontal balding became evident during his early twenties.

Language would play a unique role in Ignaz's life. Living in the heterogeneous Austro-Hungarian Empire, where eleven major languages flourished, the youthful Ignaz was exposed daily to the three most popular, Hungarian, Latin, and German. In the more rarified air of academic discourse, scientific and learned citizens still relied on Latin. At the time of Ignaz's youth, German was the language of commerce, education, and the military, while informal Hungarian remained the main language of the street. Hungarian, as a non-romance language, originated, along with the people who spoke it, mainly in the Urals, the mountain range separating Europe from Asia. With its plethora of C, Z, and S combinations, the language is so devoid of familiar syllables to the Western-trained reader that it leaves him grasping for some recognizable combination of syllables and phrases. Its pronunciation is similarly formidable. Relatively few people outside of Hungary have any facility with the language. As a consequence, medical literature of the 1800s was rarely read or even comprehensible outside of the country.

Hungarian students typically studied German supplemented by their native language but, unfortunately, in this poor province, they purportedly mastered neither. Ignaz grew up speaking Swabian German, a dialect of Eastern Europe, as his primary language. With its unusual pronunciations and peculiar phrasings, the Swabian dialect made conversations with outsiders more labored and difficult to understand. Even in this modern day, speakers of formal High German reportedly find the Swabian dialect challenging. Until his dying day, Semmelweis's heavily accented speech, complete with unusual phrasings, immediately identified his origins. For a career in which language and public rhetoric would loom critical, his linguistic foundations were less than ideal. Although Ignaz must have been sensitive very early in life to his accent and poor linguistic grounding, it was not until specialty training that he openly expressed not only "an innate aversion to everything that could be called writing," but to general polemics as well—aversions that would exert a major negative impact on his later life.[4]

Ignaz's immersion in multiple languages and ethnicities was but a linguistic microcosm of the Austro-Hungarian Empire itself, a polyglot of ethnicities, which included Bohemians, Moravians, Croats, Serbians, Hungarians, Czechs, and other smaller groups, including gypsies. Each group fiercely identified with its own native language and ethnicity, not with national boundaries agreed upon by some impersonal international commission. After the Ottoman Turks were driven out of the area in the 1500s, ministerial authorities, hoping to fill that gigantic Turkish vacuum with a more homogenized Teutonic citizenry, actively encouraged the immigration of German colonists into the less-settled eastern provinces. Of course, the opposite happened. Instead of Germans creating converts to their ways, they more commonly assimilated into the culture in which they had settled. The Semmelweis family was no exception. Although genetically German, all family members throughout their lives considered themselves Hungarian, by birth, temperament, and education.[5]

Ignaz attended Roman Catholic schools in Budapest, where he consistently excelled academically. After graduating in 1837, second in his large high school class at the Catholic gymnasium, he enrolled in the School of Law at the University of Vienna. His father had advised him that a career as a military judge would be not only intriguing but could provide a comfortable income as well. However, it took but a few weeks of lectures before Ignaz realized his colossal mistake. He found the study of law to be extremely dry and boring. One evening some medical school friends purportedly smuggled him into the hospital morgue, an old rifle manufactory, to observe a demonstration by the celebrated anatomist, Professor Baron Josef von Berres. With the students sitting on the front of their seats in anticipation, aides lifted the dripping cadaver from its smelly tub, placing it on a marble slab just as Professor Berres made his grand entrance. Despite Ignaz's initial repulsion at the putrefactive stench filling the room, he became so transfixed by the vivid display of human parts that the evening proved transformative for him.[6] Realizing that he could never go back to the study of law, Ignaz soon changed both his major and his school.

For the next two years (1838–1840) he pursued medical courses at the University of Pest. Then, in the fall of 1841, he returned to the University of Vienna. As the center of art, music, medicine, and politics, Vienna was the only place to be. The university also afforded greater professional advantages, since its graduates could practice anywhere that they wished within the Austro-Hungarian Empire. Graduates outside of Austria, on the other hand, had to limit their practices to the province from which they graduated. It was during this early Vienna era that Semmelweis joined an enclave of other young Hungarians, mostly students drawn to the excitement of Vienna and the university. Ignaz felt most at home with this group of students who all shared a common culture and language. Despite this general bonding, there was something uniquely different about Ignaz. His speech made him stand out. Close friends would often tease him good naturedly about the way he talked. Ignaz revealed his self-deprecating sense of humor, on occasion, by deliberately mispronouncing a word or coining a particularly awkward phrase. He could enjoy a laugh at his own expense as readily as did his friends.

Another medical student in the group, Lajos Markusovsky, was two years senior to Ignaz. "Marko," as friends called him, was destined to a distinguished career both in Hungarian surgery and medical journalism. The two became lifelong comrades-in-arms. Marko later provided an interesting insight, a particular sensitivity, to his friend's personality. Although Ignaz generally got along well with people, he could be easily slighted, even angered, by a comment offered by someone in complete innocence. But, once the "slight" had been fully explained to him, he could forgive just as readily as he had been offended.[7] As a faithful supporter of Semmelweis and his work, Marko often served as his mouthpiece at various points in his career.

"Prodrome"

When Ignaz enrolled in Vienna's medical school, he was naively entering a tumultuous political and scientific atmosphere that, at his young age of twenty-three, he could not even begin to comprehend. Medical theory was still dominated by medievalism. In fact, the roots of Semmelweis's future nineteenth-century vexations could be traced back, incredibly, two thousand years, to the medical theories propounded by Hippocrates around 400 BCE. Hippocrates considered the ultimate cause of diseases to be so inscrutable that they were beyond all human comprehension. Disease resulted from some mysterious interaction between the environment and an individual's constitution—a consequence of a patient's bodily functions interacting with the atmosphere and a climate shaped by "heavenly spheres." In one of his classics, *Airs, Waters and Places*, Hippocrates claimed that astronomy contributed to medicine in a large way. Indeed, "knowledge of the rising and the setting of the stars, which include the planets . . . and of the seasons, the winds, the Moon, Sun and stars will allow the physician to succeed best in securing health and will achieve the greatest triumphs in the practice of his art."[8] Believing that treatment should be both gentle and simple, Hippocrates espoused baths and poultices, purgatives and emetics, bloodletting and rest in a supportive environment.

Thomas Sydenham

With the passage of millennia and the fading of memories, medical practitioners eventually strayed widely from the teachings of Hippocrates. As a consequence, when a soon-to-be famous London physician, Thomas Sydenham, began his practice centuries later, in the mid-1600s, medicine had degenerated into a general state of chaos, rudderless, possessing no organized or rational system for understanding how diseases form in the body. Treatment regimens of that era were no better, consisting of little more than the irrational and blunderbuss offerings of herbal concoctions and heavy metals to the suffering patient.[9] Sydenham was so distressed by the disordered medical theorizing he encountered that he began fighting for change, determined to reinstate Hippocrates's humoralist theories. In fact, during his career, he earned the title "The English Hippocrates," because of his espousal of Hippocratic principles, plus his encyclopedic knowledge.

How could Sydenham's life connect, in a negative way, to a young Semmelweis two hundred years later? Those archaic Hippocratic beliefs would prove nearly as immutable as the six-hundred-year-old walls fortifying the medieval parts of Vienna, frustrating anyone who might be inspired to introduce modern thought into medicine. Although Sydenham died in 1689, 150 years before Ignaz even entered medical school, the elder's doctrines still dominated medical theory, not just in Vienna but in the entire Western world. On a

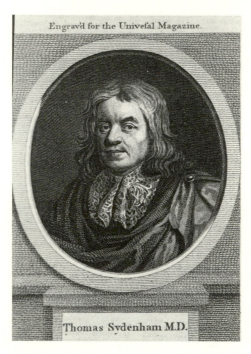

Engrav'd for the Univefal Magazine.

Thomas Sydenham M.D.

Figure 4. Thomas Sydenham (1624–1689), "The English Hippocrates" and humoralist, who introduced the *Genius* theory of disease causation. Courtesy of the US National Library of Medicine.

more positive side, Ignaz was enrolling in a school in which, a mere decade earlier, a troika of young and dynamic Viennese faculty members had begun challenging the staid hierarchies of the older medical establishment. In 1840, Ignaz would blithely enter that maelstrom, ignorant of it all.

As Sydenham gained influence, he introduced a new, empiric approach to the study of disease, while laying the foundation of clinical bedside medicine at the same time. He put little faith in pathology, the study of anatomical changes wrought by disease. To him, studying dead tissues and organs in the morgue was not the best use of time. Observing diseases in the living being, as they developed, offered a more fruitful approach. By keeping detailed records of all information he extracted at the bedside, Sydenham began building profiles of diseases based upon their method of presentation. Diseases could manifest themselves in a variety of ways, such as skin rashes, convulsions, paralyses, or distinct fevers. If viewed carefully in their proper combinations, these signs and symptoms could often paint a unique and accurate picture of a particular disease.

As his work progressed, Sydenham not only better defined diseases already known to exist, but he also identified some new ones, such as scarlet fever and the eponymous Sydenham's Chorea (Saint Vitus Dance), a complication of rheumatic fever. Each disease chronicled by Sydenham displayed certain morbid patterns of physical signs, symptoms, and clinical courses that proved to be consistent from person to person suffering with that disease. He knew that whatever underlying biological principles needed to produce those morbid patterns had to be consistent in each and every victim of the disease. It prompted him to pronounce that "the selfsame phenomena that you would observe in the sickness of a Socrates you would observe in the sickness of a simpleton."[10] Diseases, like all other natural phenomena, should be readily classifiable, much like Linnaeus had done with the plant kingdom.[11] More importantly, these classification schemes should yield great insights into how physicians should treat diseases—the ultimate reason for studying diseases. Sydenham brought an organized approach to diagnosis. On first sight it seemed rational, almost modern. So what principles did Sydenham champion that would prove so problematic to a young Semmelweis?

Genius

As Sydenham meticulously studied a wide range of maladies, from fevers to exanthems (skin eruptions), inflamed throats to confusional states, he searched for some underlying universal process of disease causation, some mechanism common to all maladies, that might explain how diseases originated and propagated within the populace. Toiling in the 1600s, in an environment generally bereft of science, Sydenham theorized, much as Hippocrates had, that certain ill-defined forces of nature must exist in common for all such diseases. Building upon the theories of Hippocrates, he employed the term "*Genius*" to describe such transcendent or metaphysical forces of nature. By definition, such etiological forces were so complex as to defy human understanding—so inexplicable that even someone possessing a full understanding of all principles of contemporary science would still be unable to elucidate their nature. He imagined these forces to be in a constant state of flux, like roiling clouds in the high atmosphere or broiling stews emanating from caldrons deep within the bowels of the earth. According to Sydenham's scheme, this *Genius* force exerted its energy causing diseases to materialize along one of two different pathways: *Genius dyscrasis* or *Genius epidemicus*.

Genius Dyscrasis

Sydenham was most concerned with the troublesome febrile ill-nesses that were so ubiquitous within the London citizenry. Per his humoralist notions, he recognized each of the commonly accepted humors of that era, such as phlegm and gall, both yellow and black, and the special one—blood. He was convinced that bodily fluids—that is, the juices, not the solids—were the important regulators of both health and disease. "The blood no question is the great genius of the body, and that which is most concerned in the nourishment, health and sickness of the man. . . . the blood, I say, that is so much concerned almost in every disease."[12]

By Sydenham's reckoning, disease resulted when any of the bodi-ly fluids, blood in particular, transformed from a normal to a patho-logic state. It might present as gout, skin eruptions, inflammation of the tissues, pneumonia, and so on. But degeneration, or dyscrasia, of the blood was the one element common to each manifestation. In Semmelweis's time, this dyscrasia was recognized as a "sepsis," or infection, of the blood, even though the term infection lacked any connection to bacterial contamination. Treatment was obvious: reduce the excess humors.

Genius Epidemicus

Sydenham also studied the contagions, a more highly infectious group of diseases, such as smallpox or cholera, that resulted in ep-idemic fevers. In his celebrated book, *De Febris*, Sydenham, like Hippocrates, again linked such great epidemics to the weather, claiming that contagious fevers arose as a result of meteorological phenomena, "some unknown constitution of the atmosphere; this arises from a miasma due partly to 'the exhalations of the sick and of the corpses of those dead of the disease.'"[13] "By the effluvia from these," he contended, "the atmosphere becomes contaminate, and the bodies of men are predisposed and determined, as the case may be, to this or that complaint."[14]

This *Genius* force, the *G. epidemicus*, resided not in the bowels of the earth like *G. dyscrasis*, but rather within the heavens or the stratosphere. Puerperal fever could have been included in the group of "non-epidemic fevers," those that emanate from the "bowels of the earth," or, just as easily, in the "epidemic fevers," dependent upon meteorological phenomena. With time, physicians identified puerperal fever as residing within the epidemic fever group, since its incidence did wax and wane inexplicably. To give physicians guidance as they diagnosed and treated their patients' illnesses, Sydenham initiated what would become a centuries-long tradition by urging them to keep detailed meteorological records.

John Locke, physician and philosopher, who became acquainted with Sydenham midway through the latter's career, ultimately served to extend Sydenham's teachings well beyond England. Locke was so enamored of Sydenham's methods that he referred to him as "the great genius of physic." As the senior man's apprentice and sometime amanuensis, it was Locke who convinced Sydenham to write his two most enduring works, *Observationes Medicae* and *De Febris* (fevers).

Herman Boerhaave

After Sydenham's death in 1689, Locke began spreading his teacher's doctrines to most of the major medical figures of Europe, including one Herman Boerhaave, professor of physik in Leyden. It was Boerhaave, more than any other figure in medicine, who greatly extended Sydenham's observations and influence a generation after the latter's death.[15] As a consequence, the Sydenham brand of humoralism became densely interwoven into the fabric of medical theory throughout the Western world.

Like Sydenham, the younger Boerhaave gained great prominence in the world of medicine a generation later. In fact, many medical historians consider him to be the most distinguished person in the entire history of Western medicine.[16] So gifted a lecturer and bedside teacher was Boerhaave that his reputation and influence even-

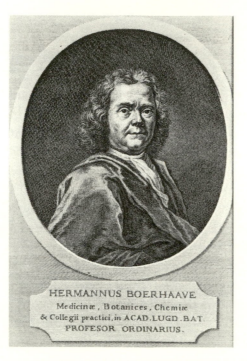

HERMANNUS BOERHAAVE
Medicinæ , Botanices , Chemiæ
& Collegii practici, in ACAD.LUGD .BAT.
PROFESOR ORDINARIUS.

Figure 5. Herman Boerhaave (1668–1738), noted Dutch physician whose book, *Aphorisms*, formed an important part of the University of Vienna's nineteenth-century medical curriculum. Courtesy of the US National Library of Medicine.

tually eclipsed even that of Sydenham. According to one apocryphal tale, he enjoyed, at his height, such renown that a Chinese Mandarin, hoping to communicate with the doctor, addressed a letter to "The Great Dr. Boerhaave, Europe." It was reportedly delivered in a timely manner.[17] Students from all over continental Europe, Britain, Russia, and as far away as America descended upon Leyden to study under the master. Many of his new graduates returned to their respective homelands, where they established medical schools espousing the Boerhaavian method.

As he lectured and practiced over the years, Boerhaave acquired vast quantities of information concerning all aspects of medicine. It seemed only natural that he share his wealth of information with the world. In 1709, he distilled his many observations into a book designed for both student and practitioner, *Aphorisms Concerning the Knowledge and Cure of Diseases*, a 500-page tome comprised of 1,500 observational verities gained through his lifetime in medicine. Although Boerhaave died in 1738, his influence, like Sydenham's, lived on in his publications and in the lives of his former students.

Although the theories of Sydenham and Boerhaave made sense

in the minds of practicing physicians in this non-scientific era, the problem arose when these theories failed to evolve with time. By the end of the eighteenth century, they had become hopelessly anachronistic. To the orthodox physician of the 1800s, still ignorant about the world of bacteria, the *Genius* factor remained critical to their manner of theorizing. Diseases were not caused by a single agent or factor. They resulted from multifactorial causes—not just *Genius dyscrasis* or *epidemicus*, although they were the two principle causes. Other influences entered in, such as the patient's nutritional or psychological state, or even such elusive, ill-defined conditions as a wounded sense of modesty, emotional embarrassment, and so on. As combinations of these factors interacted, full-blown disease eventuated from a perfect storm of concomitant forces. Two patients suffering with identical signs and symptoms might well be diagnosed with entirely different ailments, since so much depended on climatic variables and the patients' individual constitutions. Only in obvious epidemic conditions, such as the plague or cholera, did physicians diagnose the same illness in multiple individuals presenting contemporaneously with nearly identical signs and symptoms.

Since the humoralist physician was most concerned with the patient's constitution and the metaphysical forces involved, once he was confident that he understood those factors, the bulk of his diagnostic efforts was over. Viewing the body holistically, he was naturally less concerned than was the anatomic pathologist with physical manifestations within organ systems. Whether or not a liver or heart was enlarged was of less importance in his heuristic scheme. Performing a physical exam was almost anti-climactic. It typically consisted of little more than placing his hand to the forehead, inspecting the surface of the protruded tongue, and holding a full glass of urine up to the light. If he suspected diabetes, he might taste the urine to assess its sugar content. That was it.

Heroic Therapy

Since medicine lacked a scientific base, treatment methods were still based upon the humoral doctrines of Sydenham and Boerhaave, involving more art than science. Every cure was said to involve "a set of determinative values for a fixed number of variables."[18] These variables included: type of treatment, its intensity, the stage of disease at which it was applied, and the duration of time in which the treatment would be rendered.[19] One could judge a physician's value as an artisan by how adroitly he formulated the ideal treatment regimen—a mental exercise matching the multiple facets of treatment against those presented by the disease. In theory, the closer that opposing facets fit together, the more effective would be the treatment. Still, only so many therapeutic options were at the physician's disposal. Bloodletting, the most dangerous, was also the most popular. But one could just as well employ sweating; urination; purging; emetics; clysters (enemas); or the use of setons, that is, ligatures drawn into and out of the skin by needles. If left in place for days, pus inevitably issued from both sites, where the seton entered and exited the skin. Humoralists saw such purulent emanations as humors escaping from both portals. The seton was working—doing what it was supposed to be doing. Despite their lack of scientific merit, such primitive treatments were widely employed by treating physicians. Not only were such measures taxing to the patient, they proved fatal all too frequently. Such was heroic therapy, still thriving, anachronistically, in the culture of medicine more than 150 years after Sydenham's death in 1689.

Therapeutic Nihilism

A smaller, generally more enlightened segment of the physician community remained more inherently skeptical of the humoral doctrine and the treatment methods it implied. Sticking to their principles, they refused to treat patients with such drastic methods, relying more on natural processes, such as rest, clean air, and healthy diet. These were the therapeutic nihilists. One had to be, ironically, heroic to adhere to such a position. If a patient were deteriorating before the physician's very eyes, it required strong convictions on his part to continue with a regimen of little more than bed rest and clean air. In the event of a patient death, those physicians who treated heroically could at least be absolved from fault. After all, they had done everything humanly possible to save the patient. Not so with the therapeutic nihilist. He risked the legal or physical wrath of surviving family members.

Gerard Van Swieten

In 1740, when Maria Theresa assumed the Austro-Hungarian throne, these archaic methods of medical theorizing, diagnosing, and treating were in full flower. Maria Theresa's accomplishments during her forty year reign were many. She centralized Habsburg powers into Vienna's Schonbrunn Palace. As a product of the Enlightenment, she pursued many benevolent social reforms, such as improving the health of all her subjects and providing aid to the poverty-stricken masses. As a mother of sixteen children, she felt a special affinity for the thousands of unmarried Viennese women, poor, pregnant, virtually bereft of any maternity care, and all too often abandoned. One of her grand plans consisted of building a general hospital dedicated to the poor. Just as she employed a prime minister to prosecute her general objectives, she desired to hire a physician, a protomedicus, to similarly execute her medical projects. In 1745, after a prolonged search, she found her man in Dutchman Gerard van Swieten, committed humoralist and star protégé of the great Herman Boerhaave of Leyden.

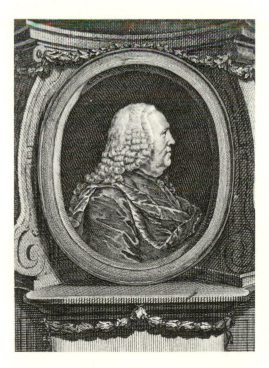

Figure 6. Gerard van Swieten (1700–1772), Boerhaave's protégé, who brought his form of humoralism to Vienna. Courtesy of the US National Library of Medicine.

As protomedicus, van Swieten served as the empress's personal physician. He had three other positions, as well—director and executor of public health, overseer of medical school curriculum, and chief of the Vienna medical faculty. His humoralist approach to medical theory was further fortified when another student of Boerhaave, Anton DeHaen, joined van Swieten nine years later, to serve as director of the Vienna Clinic. Since both men lived well into the late 1700s, they exercised near-dictatorial power over medical education for nearly thirty years. Not surprisingly, the two men imported the best known doctrines of their era—those of their renowned mentor, Boerhaave. His esteemed theories, still relevant in the 1750s, seemed a perfect fit for the empress's aims. Joining the teaching methods of Sydenham's, already in existence for a generation, Boerhaave's humoral theories became the central part of Vienna's curriculum. After Maria Theresa's death in 1780, her son, Franz Joseph, (Joseph II) assumed the throne. Continuing his mother's benevolent social programs, he finally brought her vision to fruition, in 1784, by converting an almshouse for old soldiers into the Vienna General Hospital (Allegemeine Krankenhaus). Built just outside the old fortifying walls of the city, the gigantic, three story hospital, Europe's largest, accommodated a total of two thousand patients, with male and female wards dedicated to both internal medicine and surgery. Here the poor and disaffected could receive the care and attention they so badly needed.

Even the insane had their space in this facility. The looming Narrenturm, or "Tower of Fools," can be seen in the center background. This cylindrical, five-story insane asylum, where all inmates were sequestered behind locked doors, chained to the walls in their individual cells, was nothing more than a prison for the insane. More pertinent to the interests of Semmelweis, the ministry had also allotted a similarly large maternity wing, containing two hundred beds, within the facility, dedicated to the care of gravid, impecunious, single young women.

Around century's end, a confusing succession of emperors and protomedicae ensued, consequent to some premature royal deaths and a chaotic political state in central Europe brought about by the Napoleonic wars. Although Gerard van Swieten died in 1772, his considerable influence lasted beyond that time. For the new brand

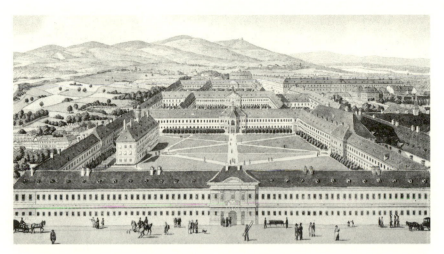

Figure 7. The massive Vienna General Hospital where Semmelweis researched and developed his theory of puerperal fever causation. Courtesy of Vienna University's Josephinum.

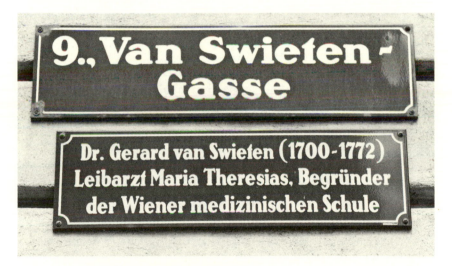

Figure 8. A current street sign near the University of Vienna Medical School named in honor of Gerard van Swieten. The inscription indicates that van Swieten was both personal physician to Maria Theresa and founder of the medical school. Photograph by Theodore G. Obenchain.

of medicine van Swieten had bestowed upon Austria, the city of Vienna named a street in his honor, still in existence today near the medical school.

Joseph II died in 1790 and was succeeded, ultimately, in 1792, by

Franz II (who later became Franz I), beginning a reign that would last until 1835. Through it all, edicts from the offices of the ministry and protomedicus remained consistently repressive. Virtually all social measures emanating from Schonbrunn Palace were enacted not so much on their inherent merits as through the simple emotion of fear. The majority of repressive medical policies during those years were a direct reflection of the views espoused by the ministry and the protomedicus.

In 1796, imperial authorities appointed the next protomedicus of consequence, Joseph Andreas Stifft, a man who proved to be just as influential in his position as van Swieten had been. Since Stifft held office until his death in 1836, his policies held sway for another forty years. Generations of young physicians-to-be were thus indoctrinated in the same medieval theories that had by now become hopelessly anachronistic even as Semmelweis, the young medical student, appeared on the scene.

Restoration Program

By the end of the eighteenth century, nearly fifty years before Semmelweis, two new theories arose that challenged the humoralist status quo. The first, Brunonianism, was named after its creator, John Brown, of Edinburgh. The theory, with its reference to the existence of ill-defined excitable forces residing within the body, was merely a newer, more modern iteration of humoralism. The second new theory was the anatomic discipline called neuroanatomy, the pioneering new science of Franz Joseph Gall. Both schemes became increasingly popular, especially among Vienna's medical elite. In a zero sum game, the theories of Brown and Gall had become ascendant at the expense of those of Sydenham and Boerhaave. But to the ministerial hierarchy, Brown's and Gall's new theories were viewed as nothing but spin-offs of ideas engendered through the intellectual and secular spirit of the French Revolution. As such, they were not only too materialistic, but they ran counter to contemporary religious principles as well. The emperor, fully supported by Stifft, set his public policy under the guidance of his own dictum, "Stick with the positive! Honor that which is ancient! The ancient is good. I want no musing."[20] Openly hostile to any and all scientific innovation, both men monitored such curricular developments nervously, waiting for a propitious time to reverse these worrisome changes.

In the early years of 1800, the two decided to act, instituting a formal Restoration Program, aimed at returning to the valued traditional theories of old, prior to the French Revolution.[21] As a result of this program, three events took place in the early nineteenth century that would foreshadow Semmelweis's own fate a half century later. The first victim was Vienna's own Leopold Auenbrugger, originator of a bedside diagnostic technique called percussion. The atmosphere in Vienna had become so hostile to medical innovation that Auenbrugger was forced to flee to the more receptive environment of Paris in order to continue his work.[22] Formalizing the ministerial position, Stifft next prohibited any and all lectures on Brunonianism and neuroanatomy, viewing both disciplines in the same light as percussion. All such theories were considered full-out confrontations against the medical establishment, tantamount to an open declaration of war on all humoralist doctrine. In 1804, with all avenues of discourse blocked by such autocratic ministerial edicts, Joseph Frank, the Viennese leader of Brunonianism, escaped to Paris, like Auenbrugger, with Gall following one year later. Nor would this repressive atmosphere dissipate anytime soon.

Not yet fully satisfied, Stifft further expanded the Restoration Program by reinstating traditional humoralism back into the medical curriculum. Any and all contemporary textbooks that he considered inimical to the traditionalist views of the empire were replaced with texts espousing the older tried and true theories. Once again Sydenham's and Boerhaave's views were established as gospel, especially Boerhaave's *Aphorisms Concerning the Knowledge and Cure of Diseases*.[23] Students were once again taught that *Genius epidemicus* and *Genius dyscrasis* were the major factors in disease causation.[24] Even as late as 1848, the aforementioned American professor Charles Meigs, of Jefferson University, expressed his humorist faith by observing, "Dr. Sydenham showed long ago that a condition of the atmosphere may exert modifying influences upon the nature of diseases, and, that as the constitution changes from time to time, so will the characteristic qualities of any disease undergo conformable modifications from year to year."[25] Words like *Genius*, or the all-inclusive term "cosmic-atmospheric-telluric," seemed to cover all imagined metaphysical forces of causation. Those incessant fevers, in all their forms, that plagued the citizenry were explainable by one or several facets of that term.

With the Restoration Program firmly in place, it became virtually impossible for any new, competing theories to arise, let alone flourish, no matter how well reasoned or compelling they might be. In a country like Austria that already trailed France in medical education, such a repressive environment only further exacerbated the problem. While French students worked at the bedside learning clinical medicine directly from patients, Austrians sat in the library committing medieval theory to memory. At the same time, directors of the Vienna Clinic continued amassing weather data, dutifully gathering all the proper paraphernalia for recording temperature, wind direction and velocity, barometric pressure, dew points, and the like, still hopeful that such information would help them gain new insights into disease causation. With humoralism reestablished, it is not surprising that pathological anatomy was relegated to a position subordinate to humoralism. The effects of Restoration ideology continued, ensuring that *Genius dyscrasis* and *epidemicus* would remain firmly entrenched in Austrian medicine for decades to come.[26] This entrenchment, persisting a half century later, would cause great headaches for a young Semmelweis.

Then, in 1824, a young man from Prague entered Vienna to enroll as a medical student at the university. His early and unhappy encounter with the school's system of medical education would begin a long and tortuous road of study and confrontation. Those antiquated theories imposed by Vienna's Education Ministry were about to be challenged.

Old School; New School

Karl Rokitansky, twenty-year-old student from Bohemia, enrolled in Vienna's School of Medicine fresh from three years of philosophical studies at the University of Prague. Despite his youth and fragile, chronically melancholic state, it took little time before his independent spirit was roused by the learning methods imposed by the Vienna faculty.[1]

Aphorisms

With the effects of the Restoration still holding sway, medical students were forced to contend with Boerhaave's aforementioned *Aphorisms Concerning the Knowledge and Cure of Diseases*. This 500-page distillation of his many observations was still in use in 1824, 116 years after its initial 1709 publication date. Students were not only expected to commit all 1,500 aphorisms to memory, but if they wished to pass their final exams, they had to regurgitate them on command, as well. As a carrot designed to encourage learning, those students who best memorized such aphorisms were celebrated as "eminent." Under Stifft's influence, Boerhaave's treatise, already a classic, enjoyed such dubious acceptance that it lived on, going through multiple editions and translations into numerous languages.[2] Although Boerhaave's views may have been relevant, even groundbreaking, for the 1700s, perusal of the book reveals just how antiquated his views had become by the 1820s. One major section of the book, "Diseases of the Simple Solid Fibre," included "Stiff and Elastic Fibres; Weak and Lax Fibres; Disease of the Strong and

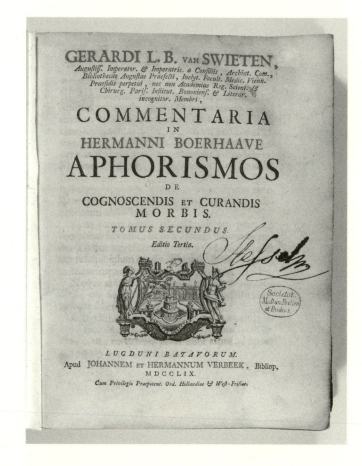

Figure 9. Gerard van Swieten's personal copy of Boerhaave's
Aphorisms. Courtesy of the Semmelweis Museum,
Budapest.

Stiff Bowels," and so on. In reading but a small part of *Aphorisms*,
such as "Of the Cold Fit in Fevers" (aphorism #621), one of the mer-
cifully shorter selections, one gains a sense of how the more enlightened Rokitansky had to have viewed such a publication: "The
Cold which happens in the beginning of acute Fevers supposeth a
less attrition of the Liquors against each other and their Vessels; a
stagnation of the Liquids at the extremities; a less contraction of the
Heart, a less quantity of Blood forced out of it; and the animal spirits
flowing less from the Cerebellum to it."[3]

Rokitansky, wondering why any nineteenth-century student

should be required to memorize even one of these sacred observations, began researching medical literature on his own, becoming largely self-taught. Reaching back nearly one hundred years, he discovered the visionary teachings of two pathologists, Giovanni Morgagni, who began the field of anatomic pathology at mid-century, and Xavier Bichat, a French pathologist at century's end. In 1761, Morgagni published *De Sedibus et Causis Morborum per anatonem indagatis* (Of the Sets and Causes of Diseases Investigated Through Anatomy), establishing anatomical pathology as a formal science. Both Morgagni and Bichat were revolutionaries in their respective countries, Italy and France, building their science upon hard facts rather than metaphysical musings. Rokitansky patterned his own investigative methods after them. As a student of Schopenhauer, Rokitansky had his spiritual side, but, like his scientific progenitors, when it came to the science of medicine, he was a strict materialist. When observing natural phenomena, he used reason alone to draw his conclusions.[4] Facts must be both immutable and reproducible. In 1827, one year before earning his medical degree, Rokitansky became an unpaid apprentice in pathology, a position with near limitless potential. Unlike France, all patient care in Austria was centralized at Vienna's General Hospital. Large numbers of patients from all over the country streamed to Vienna to receive their care there—and it was there that they died. Vienna's morgue handled in excess of three thousand autopsies annually. It took Rokitansky no time to recognize the rich research opportunity this wealth of pathology afforded him. In this era in which humoralism reigned, pathology was its poor cousin, suffering in relative obscurity. Rokitansky's mentor in pathology, Dr. Johann Wagner, although a questionable theoretician, was a superb dissector. He could allegedly un-roof an entire human bony spine in five minutes. Rokitansky took full advantage by learning Wagner's dissecting skills, eventually not only equaling him technically, but completely eclipsing him as a theoretician.

As the years passed, Rokitansky collected autopsy findings, categorized them, and correlated his findings with the patients' medical histories and physical manifestations. With time, he began to see certain disease patterns emerging from the autopsy table that matched well with images painted by patients as they described their symptoms.[5] Any patient experiencing crushing chest pain ra-

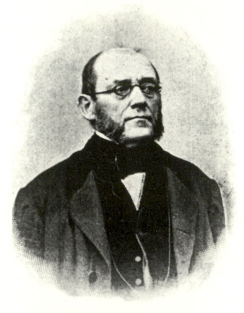

Figure 10. Karl Rokitansky
(1804–1878), revolutionary
pathologist and founder of
Vienna's New School. Courtesy
of the US National Library of
Medicine.

diating down his left arm, at autopsy, always exhibited sclerosis in
his coronary arteries. Or, the woman with a swollen and paralyzed
left arm and an ulcerating cancer in her breast, had, on autopsy, infiltration of the cancer into her nerve plexus. As Rokitansky began
collecting, correlating, and classifying his data, he recognized that
all diseases become established within the living body through identifiable and predictable, step-by-step processes. Through such methods, he developed a unique, avant-garde school of thought.

This methodology became Rokitansky's system of pathology, and
he produced prodigiously. In 1836, the same year that the repressive
Stifft died, Rokitansky published treatises in the *Medical Yearbooks
of the Imperial Royal Austrian State* covering a variety of subjects
as diverse as intestinal pathology, rupture of the aorta, aspects of
new bone formation, and duplication of the uterus. As certain professors of medicine and other authorities read his work, they immediately recognized the "particularly logical spirit" and the impressive original language used by the author. These essays, so different
in content and clarity from almost anything produced before, gave
clear evidence of a new way of thinking. A new school of medicine
thus emerged with Karl Rokitansky as its father and his autopsy slab

in the dead house of the Vienna General Hospital, its epicenter. This humble origin marked the beginning of one of the most celebrated and illustrious eras not only in the history of Vienna's School of Medicine, but of the world as well.[6]

Rokitansky was an extraordinary worker. During the course of his career he personally performed over thirty thousand autopsies. He organized and published his massive body of information in three volumes, the *Handbook of Pathologic Anatomy*, printed between 1842 and 1846. His work, subsequently translated into multiple languages, soon became a classic, used by students the world over.

Rokitansky was also a venerated teacher of medical students and physicians specializing in the newly evolving field of anatomic pathology. With his heavily accented speech, the professor was difficult to understand, yet his dry wit and genial manner made his lectures and demonstrations compelling. Medical students crowded the lecture halls whenever he lectured.[7] Rokitansky made his presentations more vivid and memorable by the liberal use of similes. He might describe an abnormal sludge in the gall-bladder as "anchovy paste," while "raspberry-jam" filled a hemorrhagic cyst, or "coffee-grounds" brown residue occupied the stomach.[8]

While the practical implications of Rokitansky's new scientific method were enormous, his approach was necessarily limited to the morgue. As a pathologist, his work locus was the dead house, not the bedside. If his new scientific method were to progress further, Rokitansky's advances would need to be incorporated into clinical, that is, bedside medicine. Practicing physicians would require a practical way to diagnose, at the bedside, changes wrought by disease in the living, ailing human being. The man who would fulfill that need was Josef Skoda, the second man in the New School triumvirate. He would become so effective in the development of those bedside methods that he could ultimately detect physical changes months before they were discoverable on the autopsy table. Once Skoda fully developed his art, it dovetailed beautifully with Rokitansky's laboratory science.

Skoda had been raised in such poverty in Bohemia that, to enter medical school, he spent six days walking the two hundred miles from Prague to Vienna, arriving in 1827, three years after Rokitansky. As Skoda was confronted with the same curricular require-

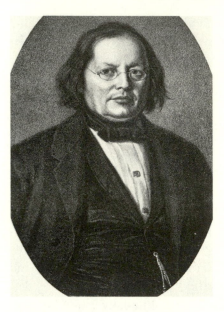

Figure 11. Josef Skoda (1805–1881),
iconic developer of scientific
diagnostic bedside techniques and
principle mentor to Semmelweis.
Courtesy of the US National Library
of Medicine.

ments, memorizing meaningless, archaic theory, he rebelled and
began studying on his own, another autodidact in the Rokitansky
mold. Mathematics and physics became his guiding lights. After receiving his MD in 1831, Skoda remained at the hospital, working
as an unpaid assistant on the medical wards. It was in that environment that he began to pursue two new bedside arts of diagnosis that
would become strongly identified with him, auscultation and percussion. Both techniques had previously been banned during Vienna's Restoration Program for being too materialistic and dangerous.

Percussion

The technique of percussion was originally popularized by vintners.
By merely tapping on their oak barrels they learned to discern the
level of wine within the container. A sudden change in sound, from
high-pitched to resonant—solid to hollow—identified the wine level
within the barrel. In humans the examiner percusses by the simple
tapping of his right middle fingertip on the left middle fingertip as
the latter glides along the side of the abdomen, chest, or some other
anatomical part. A competent percussor can not only detect the borders of the underlying organ, such as the heart; he can also conclude

whether it is enlarged or of normal size—merely by its anatomic boundaries and the sounds elicited. By percussing over the chest one can as well detect whether the lung has become solidified with inflammatory tissue (pneumonia), or is perhaps covered with fluid (effusion), or collapsed by air (pneumothorax). Vienna's own afore-mentioned Leopold Auenbrugger had earlier adapted the percussive technique to medicine. In 1761, he published his experiences. Rath-er than bestowing honor on this original thinker, Vienna's medical authorities were incensed by his dangerous practices, forcing his aforementioned escape to Paris.

Auscultation

The better known auscultation became practical only after René T. H. Laennec, of Paris, invented the stethoscope in 1816. However, outside of France, it was Skoda who popularized the technique two decades later.[9] By placing the stethoscope over the heart and blood vessels, Skoda learned that he could distinguish the different sounds of vascular turbulence, equating particular sounds with certain an-atomic states, both normal and abnormal. Before Skoda, physicians had little understanding of the origin of heart sounds. He not only elucidated the normal sounds of heart contraction (systole) from re-laxation (diastole), he also identified the adventitial sounds, calling such abnormalities "murmurs."[10] As Skoda observed, "In order to make it easier to avoid any misunderstandings, I call the tick-tack of the heart and the arteries sounds, and I use the word murmur never to indicate the tick-tack, but to indicate the noises as made by a bellows, a grater, a saw, a rasp, friction noises."[11] By listening to these murmurs, Skoda learned to correlate their sound patterns with anatomic conditions, such as a leaky, incompetent heart valve, or a valve which is so scarred and narrow that it emits yet another distinctive sound of turbulence. In essence, he learned to diagnose heart conditions through percussing its expanded borders and by ausculting the abnormal sounds emitted. As Skoda gained experi-ence he extended his diagnostic acumen to other conditions within the chest, including spasm in the bronchial tubes, collapsed lung, and pneumonia, as well as other types of solidifications, such as tumors of the lung. The amount of information that Skoda could gain at the bedside merely by his careful assessment of sounds emitted from the various organs was truly remarkable.

As Skoda became highly skilled in the art of defining anatomical states through the mere use of bedside techniques, he ushered in a new era of medicine called "anatomical clinicism," the true clinical counterpart to Rokitansky's anatomical pathology.[12] Skoda refined his bedside skills by utilizing two principles. First, he relied upon rational physical principles to analyze variations of pressure waves moving through a medium, the science of vibrations. It helped him to scientifically interpret disparate types of turbulence, from the normal sounds of blood progressing through a vessel to its passage through abnormally constricted or dilated apertures. From such analyses he could form a mental picture of that constricted or dilated heart valve, or that pathologic "bruit," a sound originating from a direct, pathological connection between an artery and a vein, rather than through their usual connection via a system of capillaries.

Modus Tollens

The second tool Skoda used to help him make sense of the maze of abnormal bodily shapes and sounds was the use of a simple syllogism, *modus tollens*, or *per exclusionem*, one of those short-form scenarios of logic boiled down to near-mathematical formulations, that provide for a more rational and systematic way of arriving at the facts. While the Latin phrasing sounds impressive, the process, in plain English, is nothing more than diagnosing a disease, or arriving at the most logical scientific theory, through diagnostic exclusion, that is, by eliminating certain presented characteristics that do not fit in logically with the formulation at hand. As Skoda contemplated the different sorts of shapes, sights, and sounds with which patients presented, he had to decide which of them did, or did not, contribute to his arriving at a specific diagnosis. *Per exclusionem* in effect, helped him exclude factors that were confusing or, at least, not germane to his specific observation. Skoda originally directed his talents exclusively to diseases of the chest but, as he perfected his techniques, he made his art applicable to the entire body.[13]

After diagnosing his patients, he followed them closely, making certain to corroborate his bedside findings with what he found at the autopsy table, if and when they died. As Skoda ausculted and percussed, he learned not only to pinpoint the diagnosis but, with Rokitansky's method of pathology, to arrive at a unified understanding of the steps through which the disease developed—the first logical methodology that physicians had for gaining an understanding of the patient and his disease, all derived from a "simple" bedside encounter.

When it came to examining the ailing patient, the less-enlightened, humoralist physician looked for holistic evidence, a systemic change in his patient's physical state, such as fever or dry skin. In contrast, the new physician focused on specific organ systems, detecting perhaps an enlarged heart or liver, solidified lungs, and the like. It was the detection of diseased organ systems that was important. Such a finding could very well lend insights into whatever disease process was in play. Any young physician who learned Skoda's techniques, and truly understood their implications in light of Rokitansky's science, gained not only a specific diagnosis but also a better understanding of the disease process as well. Compared to the average clueless humoral practitioner's examination, anyone who employed the arts of percussion and auscultation literally held in his hands a revolutionary set of tools that could enable him to gain a modern understanding of disease.

In Skoda's case, he became so accomplished in his art that he seemed prescient to the less experienced observer, telling Rokitansky what the autopsy would reveal days or even months before the patient died. In 1839, a mere ten years after earning his medical degree, Skoda distilled his experience into a textbook, *Treatise on Percussion and Auscultation*—another classic emanating from the University of Vienna's New School of medicine. Despite his cold and cerebral mien as a man who tolerated no nonsense, Skoda's diagnostic talents compelled students from around the world to study under him in Vienna. But Skoda was less than universally admired. During his early career, in particular, many older physicians viewed him and his methods with suspicion. Unable to understand his new way of thinking, they sarcastically dismissed his techniques with such statements as, "the stethoscope is the true microscope of the ear through which one can hear the fleas cough."[14]

The personal Skoda was an enigma, completely indifferent to any and all social mores, tactless, possessing few if any social graces. He suffered from a similar lack of sartorial concerns, as his threadbare clothing attested.[15] Early in his career Skoda demonstrated his steely individualism when, without securing permission from his superiors, he performed an emergency tracheotomy on a man dying of acute airway obstruction. Despite clearly saving the man's life, Skoda was reprimanded for displaying an excessive level of independence. Hospital authorities banished him to work for a period of one year in the medieval Narrenturm, Vienna General's own insane asylum. Forty years had passed since Frenchman Philippe Pinel had introduced enlightenment into psychiatry by ushering in the "Moral Therapy" of mental patients. Rejecting the usual explanations of mental illness, such as one's inherent moral shortcomings, or providential retribution for one's past sins, Pinel not only ordered all mental patients at Paris's Bicetre Hospital to be unchained, but he insisted on treating them in a humane manner, as well. Unfortunately, Pinel's more enlightened attitude towards mental illness would not reach Vienna for decades, causing significant problems for mental patients of the 1830s and later for an ailing Semmelweis. Skoda made the best of his one year sentence by gaining entrance behind all locked doors, percussing and ausculting the befuddled inmates, perfecting his technique as he defined the boundaries of their internal organs.

Skoda was an inherent therapeutic nihilist. He recognized that all of the induced purging, vomiting, sweating, bloodletting, and the like were not only a waste of time, but could be dangerous. But he did distinguish between hopelessness and usefulness. If he diagnosed an abnormal collection of fluid on the lung or heart of a patient, he would aggressively drain such effusions with a needle. In the more typical case in which no definitive treatment was available, once he made his diagnosis, Skoda would walk away, leaving his acolytes to devise some treatment scheme.

Semmelweis was enormously influenced by Skoda, not only by his diagnostic genius, his method of critical reasoning, but in applying mathematics to medicine as well. It was under Skoda that Semmelweis refined his senses of induction and deduction, and learned how to think like a scientist.

Ferdinand von Hebra

The third person of this New School triumvirate, who proved important to Semmelweis's education, was Ferdinand von Hebra, a man only two years older than Semmelweis. The two became close friends. In fact, Hebra's admiration for Semmelweis became so great that he later chose the young accoucheur to attend his own wife's delivery, the greatest compliment any physician can bestow upon a colleague.[16] Hebra amazed his own students with his diagnostic acumen. As one former student later recalled, Hebra could tell what trade the person practiced merely by examining the calluses on his hands. "He is a cobbler and suffers from scabies," was but one example.[17] Hebra was as warm and ebullient as Skoda, the man under whom he began working, was dour. He could get along with anyone. Yet, were this Semmelweis tale a Shakespearean tragedy, it would be Hebra, ironically, who was destined to play the role of Marcus Brutus.

Soon after Hebra earned his Vienna medical degree in 1841, Skoda appointed him director of the "itch ward," in charge of patients suffering from various skin abnormalities. Since diseases of the skin were so poorly understood, such patients were treated as pariahs, in essence, warehoused on a ward—out of sight and out of mind. The majority of "itch ward" patients suffered from scabies, a mite infection of the skin. But the more enlightened physicians of the era did not believe that mites were the cause of such a malady. According to nineteenth-century humoralist theory, skin rashes (exanthems), including scabies, were external manifestations of a unique mix of humors—a crasis of the blood à la Sydenham. Rashes appeared and vanished concurrent with the inward and outward movement of humors through pores in the skin. Treatment consisted of "driving out the acrimonious and purifying the humors by purification of the blood."[18] In practice, this meant administering laxatives and emetics to these long-suffering patients.[19]

Hebra, doubting the validity of such a theory, set out to investigate it. After injecting a mite underneath the skin of his own left middle finger, he dutifully recorded the fluctuating changes occurring within his body, such as the local inflammatory reaction and the more generalized itching. Ultimately, he proved that scabies was

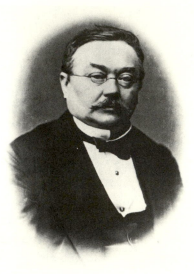

Figure 12. Ferdinand von Hebra
(1816–1880), father of modern dermatology and longtime friend of
Semmelweis. Courtesy of the US
National Library of Medicine.

nothing more than an infectious disease caused by the skin mite,
not a manifestation of some humoral crasis. By applying Rokitansky's logical approach to diseases of the skin, Hebra slowly compiled
a mass of patho-anatomic facts. He organized and classified various
conditions of the skin, bringing order to a chaotic group of diseases.[20]
In 1848, just seven years after graduation, Hebra published *Classification of Diseases of the Skin*, another medical classic.

With Rokitansky's three volumes of *Handbook of Pathologic
Anatomy*, plus the works of Skoda and Hebra, the University of Vienna had entered into its greatest era ever, surpassing Paris as the
world's new mecca of medicine. By providing a rational window into
pathological processes, how diseases developed and became manifest, the combination of Rokitansky's, Skoda's, and Hebra's methods
could be viewed as a creative unity, a method that matured into
modern clinical medicine. The trio had not only created the foundation of scientific bedside medicine, they also, like three legs of a
stool, provided a great base of stability for Vienna's New School of
medical thought.[21]

One could arguably consider Josef Kolletschka a fourth, if less
prominent, member of the New School. As a forensic pathologist,
he, like Semmelweis, spent a major part of his time in the morgue

performing autopsies. Through this shared pastime the two naturally became close friends. Kolletschka would, in his own tragically serendipitous way, make a critical and major contribution to the riddle of puerperal fever.

The advent of the New School in the 1830s was a major positive development for medicine and the suffering public. Yet, it marked the beginning of an ongoing intellectual storm within the faculty of Vienna's medical school. Semmelweis's entrance into that school in 1841 placed him in the middle of the conflict. Two clearly delineated schools of thought existed, each serving as mutual adversarial foils during this turbulent era. The first, or Old School, originally unnamed since it was the only school of thought, represented the established order, holding unquestionable control since ancient times. Like a microcosm of the larger Austrian society, adherents of the Old School placed their faith in hierarchical social schemes, the inherent or God-given right of certain individuals to rule over others. Old School members had no problem adhering to central dictatorial powers that unilaterally proscribed social, political, and economic conditions. In the case of medicine, that dictator could set the philosophical tone for the medical community by either imposing his own pet theory, such as humoralism, or by suppressing any theorizing that he considered dangerous.

Old School of Medicine

Similarly, Old School adherents considered it natural for dictators to determine curricular content and methods for testing, licensing, and the like. They resisted change by clinging to medieval ideation: disease was the result of some mystical interaction between the inner, bodily humors and the outer, cosmic and telluric (terrestrial) influences. Old School members firmly believed in heroic therapy, the vomiting, purging, sweating, heavy metal medications, and so on, that often proved worse than the disease itself. But taking the patient to the edge of mortality was the point. Unless the toxic aspects of treatment proved life-threatening, or the side effects caused some level of suffering, such treatment could hardly be considered heroic. Generally older faculty members dominated this school of thought.

Two incarnations of this group, each so important to Semmelweis's future, were Johann Klein, professor of obstetrics, and Anton Rosas, ophthalmology professor and deputy director of the medical faculty.

New School of Medicine

The second, or New School, required decades to gain ascendancy in Vienna. Once established, however, it became clear that virtually all New School tenets were antipodal to those of the Old. New School adherents were radically anti-establishment, generally opposed to central powers, including that of their own Austro-Hungarian Empire. They valued rational thought over medieval musings; material observations over metaphysics; mathematical verities, such as statistics, over intuitive correlations. To them, governmental authorities, on balance, represented a negative force in medical education. They longed for academic freedom, the ability to critically pursue their own intellectual theories. They and their colleagues, rather than ministerial authorities, should be in charge of weighing the merit of their own theories. They longed to design their own course content and to control the quality of student education. Such men were typically younger and more recently educated. Since members of the New School were rationalists, they readily recognized the danger and uselessness of contemporary treatment methods. Therapeutic nihilism was a given. As pillars of the New School, Rokitansky, Skoda, and Hebra were its personal embodiments.

It was now the mid-1840s and medical student, Ignaz Semmelweis, would bear witness to much of the scientific grandeur surrounding the New School. The influence of the New School trio on the young medical student would affect, for a lifetime, the way he formed his opinions and approached vexing clinical problems. Semmelweis would not only become the quintessential product of the New Vienna Medical School of medicine with its modern methodology, but as he struggled on with his investigative burdens, he would ultimately transcend it. But first, a word about Vienna General Hospital, the site in which Semmelweis's deliberations would incubate into a theory.

Vienna General Hospital

In 1784, decades before Semmelweis's time, benign despot Joseph II finally brought Maria Theresa's grand plan for a hospital to fruition. He converted an old soldiers' almshouse into the modern Vienna General Hospital (Allegemeines Krankenhaus), a facility in which poor citizens of Austria could receive free medical care. One section included a maternity hospital, a refuge for young mothers-to-be. Joseph II was responding to a major, longstanding social problem. Vienna, like most major European cities, was flooded with young, single expectant women, a problem that developed along with the influx of citizens from the country into the city. The first half of the nineteenth century constituted the middle of the Industrial Revolution, an era in which such inventions as the railroad, the steam engine, and the spinning jenny created new opportunities in the cities. Young women, often poorly educated, enticed by the allure of new industries, new factories, and different types of employment, traveled from their country homes into large cities like Vienna. Here they found work in factories or as domestics for affluent Viennese families. While some women, homesick, lonely, and impecunious, found solid romantic relationships in the city, others proved easy prey for any urban lothario who might be trolling the city parks and coffeehouses in search of feminine companionship. One romantic scenario played out with enough wearisome regularity to constitute a major problem not only in Vienna, but in most other large European cities, as well. As the young woman informed her mate of her delayed monthly cycle, or the doctor's confirmatory exam, too often the mate disappeared into thin air leaving her very existence threatened by her dependency and gravid state.

Alone in the city, virtually none of the young women had any family, friends, or any sort of support systems that might help care for their new charges. As a mother of sixteen children, Maria Theresa identified strongly with the plight of these women. Providing refuge to each of them was one of her major aims. Her program included a stay in Vienna's maternity wing for the final two months of a woman's pregnancy. There these young women could receive warmth, shelter, a nutritious diet, appropriate care and companionship with others similarly afflicted, all free of charge. However, with her admission, the expectant woman was entering into a social contract. Each parturient was responsible for her own housekeeping. She was, as well, required to leave the hospital within nine days after delivery, in order to make room for the next needy person. In return for the free care, for the benefit of medical science in general and medical students in particular, mothers-to-be were obliged to submit to any and all examinations by hospital staff and their students.

Such was the state of the city and the hospital in April 1844, as Ignaz Semmelweis found himself on the verge of graduation, preparing to encounter the greater world of medicine. Naturally, he began wondering about what direction his career might take in the immediate future. But before he could make any definitive career decision, his mother died unexpectedly. In what may have been the earliest indication of some peculiar facet of his personality, he departed for Pest for an entire month without bothering to first speak with any one of his faculty members. After attending his mother's services and spending time with his family, he returned to Vienna, where he received his medical degree in May. Still ruminating over career choices, he first applied to study under Skoda. Given the latter's celebrated status, however, all training positions were filled for several years into the future. Semmelweis discussed his dilemma with one of his friends, Johann Chiari, who, at the time, was an assistant in the obstetrical department. Chiari persuaded Semmelweis to pursue a short, informal trial of obstetrics under his protective wing. Semmelweis not only enjoyed the brief exposure to obstetrics, but his experience proved inspirational as well. He became intrigued by a tragic surgical case that he had shared with Chiari, a young woman with uterine fibroids. The two surgeons removed the woman's fibroid masses in an uneventful operation, only to see her die mysteriously soon after her operation. Her manner of death was highly suggestive of sepsis, a generalized infection in the bloodstream. In fact, as Semmelweis observed this woman dying with high fever and delirium, progressing to coma, it brought to mind the few young parturients that he, as a medical student, had observed deteriorating in the final stages of puerperal fever. This woman's mysterious death piqued his curiosity and became entrenched as an enigma in the back of his mind. Semmelweis enjoyed his short primer under Chiari so much that he enrolled in a formal, two-month period of instruction in obstetrics at Vienna General Hospital. That course proved so satisfying to him that he voluntarily repeated it, gaining his Master of Midwifery certificate on August 1, 1844.[1]

Sublime Versus Dark Forces

Semmelweis later described how one "sublime" aspect of obstetrics, an experience centered on a condition known as "transverse lie," helped him in choosing his career. During his four-month obstetrical course, he became proficient in the bimanual examination, a technique in which the fetal position within the uterus can be determined by applying the methods of physical examination that he had learned from his obstetrical superiors. In such an exam, one hand is placed on the abdomen overlying the dome (fundus) of the uterus while a digit or two from the other hand is placed within the birth canal. Between the two hands the examiner is able to gain a sense of the fetal position relative to the mother. With the upper, "abdominal" hand he can feel the baby's back and buttocks through the uterine fundus, while from below, his fingertips can define the position of the child's head. For a nascent therapeutic nihilist, gaining this diagnostic skill had to be empowering in itself. He could now follow the position of the fetus progressing through its various rotations in its descent through the birth canal. Not only could he now diagnose fetal position with precision, but this new skill allowed him to anticipate any upcoming fetal malrotations on a rational basis as well.

In a position called transverse lie, a child is lying in utero, with its bodily length rotated ninety degrees out of alignment, subjecting it

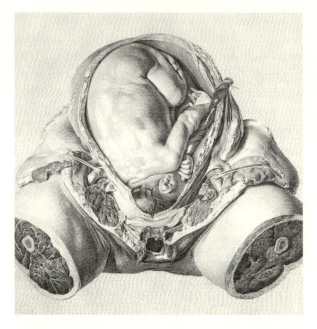

Figure 13. Copperplate engraving by Jan van Riemsdyk illustrating William Hunter's "Anatomy of the Human Gravid Uterus." Courtesy of the US National Library of Medicine.

to forces much like a tree trunk floating transversely in a river as it approaches a set of rapids. Just as the tree trunk will become stuck unless its long axis can be rotated ninety degrees into alignment with the rapids, both mother and child are similarly facing death unless the fetus can be rotated into proper alignment in a timely manner. First, the accoucheur must diagnose the problem by employing the bimanual exam. Then, to avert disaster, he must perform a simple but expert rotation of the child's body, ensuring that its length is brought into anatomic alignment with the forces within maternal birth canal—a maneuver requiring several minutes. As Semmelweis, the young novice, gained competency with this technique, he began to better appreciate the beneficent results of his fledgling efforts: disaster averted. Each success meant another healthy mother and child. This was Semmelweis's "sublime" experience, the sort of profound gratification that not only keeps one's spirits energized for the remainder of that day but, when mother and child are encountered on rounds in the days that follow, is rekindled.

Despite the positives, Semmelweis was acutely aware of a major incongruity, an imbalance, in the field of obstetrics, the sublime versus the dark side. On one hand, the accoucheur can accomplish such beneficent results with skillfully applied treatments, especially when it came to malrotations. Yet, on the dark side, in the far greater number of puerperal fever cases, "he can only offer aid that is of no avail."[2] Weighing the positives versus the negatives, to be able to rationally diagnose and treat such fetal problems as transverse lie with such gratifying results proved immensely compelling to him. On balance, the positives, the "sublime," plus the noble challenge of solving the enigma of puerperal fever, outweighed the darkness he experienced of witnessing young women dying by the score. Semmelweis had found his niche.

Assistantship

Now, with his future aspirations clear, Semmelweis could chart a more definite course. He applied for a two-year assistantship under Professor Johann Klein, director of the Department of Obstetrics at Vienna General Hospital. His application came with the enthusiastic endorsement of Chiari, who had just completed his own assistantship, plus the glowing recommendations of the New School trio. Semmelweis was profoundly disappointed when he found that the current position was already filled by a Dr. Gustave Breit. Professor Klein gave Semmelweis the choice of applying for a position elsewhere or waiting two years for Breit to complete his term. Not wishing to leave such an iconic institution that had given him such a great start, Semmelweis decided on the latter course. Accordingly, Klein appointed him to an unpaid position, "Aspirant Lecturer, and Assistant in Waiting." Since Semmelweis was still fully dependent on parental largesse, lack of remuneration did not pose any undue hardship for the new assistant in waiting.

Josefstadt

What seemed an unfortunate two-year delay for Semmelweis turned out to be, instead, a blessing in disguise. He could pursue the enigma of puerperal fever at his own pace, under his own direction.

He and close friend, Markusovsky moved into the Josefstadt section of the city adjacent to the university. Here, in Vienna's Latin Quarter, Semmelweis began two of the happiest, most carefree years

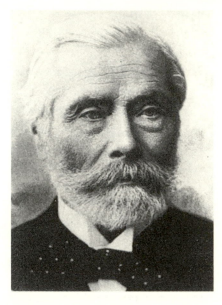

Figure 14. Lajos Markusovsky (1815–1893), prominent Hungarian surgeon, medical journalist, and longtime friend and confidant of Semmelweis.

of his life. While he had none of the pressures that accompany clinical responsibilities, he was given full access to all active clinical charts plus the most detailed and extensive departmental archives in all of Europe. His days were idyllically self-indulgent. He was free to perform autopsies in the morning, before pursuing his research for the remainder of the day. At night, he and Marko could enjoy all the pleasures that Vienna had to offer. This was the romantic era in music, and Vienna sat in its epicenter. Johann Strauss, the younger, had just made his auspicious debut in 1844, at the same time that Semmelweis was earning his medical degree. Both Strausses, senior and junior, remained friendly rivals throughout their careers. With music reputed to be elegant enough for concert venues, yet popular enough for the dance hall, father and son dominated Vienna's waltz and symphonic scene for years. As a newer form of musical expression, the waltz had just a hint of scandal associated with it. Couples, for the first time, actually embraced, instead of merely holding hands at a distance. Semmelweis, with his sudden bounty of spare time, flourished in such an environment. Friends described him as a powerful and smooth dancer. With that talent and his easy repartee, he was a natural at schmoozing with the denizens of the dance halls. He was a ladies' man. As Marko described it, "He was exceedingly popular with the ladies . . . more so than I ever was . . . . The ladies were also exceedingly popular with him. In short, he was a jolly companion, you could not wish for a better one."[3]

Despite such feminine distractions, Semmelweis pursued his primary mission sedulously. During these two years in waiting, 1844–1846, his research effort followed three informal paths: examine departmental history as revealed through its archives; review all existing, relevant theories on puerperal fever; and finally, seek enlightenment on every pathologic manifestation of puerperal fever by dissecting all patients dying on the obstetrical wards.[4] Rokitansky, as director of the Pathologic Institute, had kindly made such work available to him beginning in 1844. Over the course of nearly five years, Semmelweis performed autopsies on hundreds of puerperal fever victims, gaining great perspective on the disparate manifestations of the disease. Through his diligent pursuit of all aspects of puerperal fever, he turned these two years into something positive.

Semmelweis also broadened his general horizons by enrolling in Skoda's fifteen-month course in logic and statistics. Here Semmelweis learned the various forms of valid and invalid argumentation and how one might employ statistics to resolve particular clinical questions. He gained an understanding of the same methods of logic, especially *per exclusionem*, that had guided Skoda in the perfection of his diagnostic techniques. By emulating his mentor, Semmelweis would come to rely heavily on this new way of thinking scientifically, the method of diagnosis by exclusion—a systematic separation of wheat from chaff—as he evaluated the different theories of puerperal fever.[5]

Departmental Research

Semmelweis expended much energy investigating the history of the Obstetrics Department, which included huge stacks of medical records, extending back sixty years to the hospital's origin in 1784. Vienna General maintained some of the most detailed and accurate records in all of Europe. Digging through these records, he discovered a treasure trove of information that, along with his own pure clinical experience, had to have been most enlightening to him in his quest for the truth. Prominent in its early history was the name Johan Lucas Boer, Vienna's first obstetrician. Back in the 1880s, the Austrian ministry, anxious to improve obstetrical care in Austria, sent Johan Lucas Boer, then thirty years old, to study French and English methods for three years. Boer became so impressed with the conservative English methodology that he imported it, essentially unchanged, to the Vienna Hospital in 1789, when he assumed the chair of practical and theoretical obstetrics.

As a result of his many years of impeccable service, Boer ultimately became the first great icon of Austrian obstetrics. Eschewing active intervention, such as forceps and heroic therapy during and after labor, Boer accented, instead, the organic processes of pregnancy, generally allowing nature to follow its course under his watchful, conservative eye. He stressed healthy diets, fresh air, exercise, and normal activities as late into the pregnancy as possible.[6] Such antiquated practices as purging; using hot or ice-cold showers; and bloodletting of expectant women—a practice commonly performed to reverse their "full-bloodedness"—were terminated. Boer had an inherent distrust in the practice of using cadavers for student instruction. Instead, he employed the leather mannequin exclusively for teaching the mechanics of delivery.

During this phase of research, Semmelweis studied all aspects of puerperal fever mortality rates spanning the department's entire existence. He plotted graphs or tables contrasting rates of infection and/or mortality rates against every conceivable variable that might, in some way, be related to puerperal fever. He discovered that Boer's cumulative mortality rate in 65,000 deliveries over 33 years fluctuated, astoundingly, only a fraction above or below 1 percent. During this same era, some European clinics frequently struggled with rates exceeding 15 percent.[7] Capitalizing on his experience and exemplary record, Boer wrote *Essays Concerning Obstetrics*, a popular text designed both for practicing physicians and those in training. Boer, in general accord with his English mentors, believed that puerperal fever was in some way contagious, beginning as "a deposit in the chest or abdomen" or "a putrescence of the uterus."[8]

Anatomic Program

In 1822, just as Boer entered his thirty-third year of practice, the Ministry of Education issued a new imperative concerning anatomy: faculty members must integrate the use of cadavers into all aspects of their curriculum. Instructors in obstetrics must not only replace the mannequin with the cadaver for teaching the mechanics of delivery, but their students must also spend a major part of their time in the morgue dissecting the dead. Boer, citing his inherent reservations concerning the risks of the cadaver, refused to give up the mannequin in his teaching. Completely ignoring Boer's illustrious thirty-three year career, the ministry immediately dismissed him for insubordination. And, something that would later loom problematic for Semmelweis, the ministry replaced Boer with the aforementioned Johann Klein (fig. 15) a thirty-four-year-old man whose résumé included a mere two weeks of obstetrical training.

The politically connected Klein was a fashionable Habsburg patriot, every bit as comfortable in aristocratic as he was in medical circles. If in the company of bureaucratic superiors he knew how to ooze the requisite charm. Semmelweis supporter Dr. Franz H. Arneth, who in the 1840s became very familiar with the unctuous Klein, claimed that Klein had learned well the art of duplicity, speaking highly of a colleague in his presence, only to immediately denigrate him behind his back.[9] When it came to competence in medicine, Klein was reportedly a man of "timorous mediocrity," someone who, rather than bucking the imperial anatomic trend, enthusiastically supported the use of cadavers in medical education.[10] It took little time for Semmelweis, in his research, to discover Klein's past problems with infection. He tabulated the results, not with any malicious agenda towards Klein, but as one who conscientiously gathered data in search of the truth. As Klein concluded his first full year after succeeding Boer, his mortality rate had jumped to 7.4 percent. In the following two decades, he never came close to Boer's admirable mortality rates. While Klein at least appeared to be appropriately concerned with his high mortality rate early in his tenure, he blamed the problem on conditions such as miasmatic air, contaminated walls, *Genius epidemicus*, along with what became his favorite theory for a time, milk metastasis. Believing that any real solution lay beyond all human comprehension, it took him but a few years to settle into a state of complacent fatalism.

Had he possessed sufficient intellectual curiosity, Klein could have pursued an enigma that had existed for years within his own department, a conundrum that might have provided him with

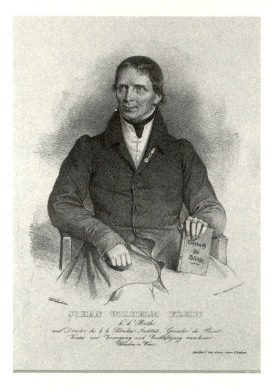

Figure 15. Lithograph of
the patrician Johann Klein,
Old School professor of obstetrics at the University of
Vienna and Semmelweis's
ultimate nemesis. By J.
Kriehuber (1831). Courtesy
of London's Wellcome
Library.

a strong clue as to the origins of puerperal fever. He ran a private
service for the wealthy and the politically connected, hermetical-
ly sealed off from the main maternity wards. No trainee was even
allowed to enter this sacrosanct spot without approval. In fact, the
ward's presence was rarely even broached in casual conversation.
Mortality rates on this special ward ran consistently around 1 percent annually. How could Klein, as he perused the monthly departmental reports, fail to notice this glaring discrepancy compared to
the epidemics raging on the charity ward? Why had he never investigated this difference? He could have easily assigned an eager
young assistant to pursue the enigma without even getting his own
hands dirty with the necessary research and dissections. But Klein,
occupying his lofty, satisfying position in life, had grown much too
comfortable. He enjoyed considerable wealth; held a prestigious university position; cared for Vienna's elite; and instructed young physicians, a position in which he could drop his pearls of wisdom to his
subordinates on daily rounds. Had he ever possessed any intellectual
curiosity at all, it had died years before.

Ward Divisions

Originally the maternity wing had 178 beds, but during the decade of the 1830s, Klein's busy department expanded, adding the eighth and ninth wards for a total bed count of 800, all within one department. Whether midwife or medical student, everyone worked within a single group. Then in 1839, the ministry mandated that students in the department be divided into two groups. Medical students were assigned exclusively to Division I, while student midwives were relegated to Division II. Patient admissions alternated between the two divisions on a daily basis.[11] As Semmelweis labored in the archives, whether he realized it or not, this split into two divisions provided him with a near-perfect randomized study. Not only were the two wards sitting adjacent to each other, differing only slightly in physical design, but patients received virtually identical treatment in each division, as well. Since all entering patients were randomly assigned to either Division I or II on alternating days, the arrangement offered him the opportunity of contrasting the two divisions.

As Semmelweis perused the records, he made an important discovery concerning infection rates. Before the split into two divisions, only one mortality rate could be reported. Although the care rendered to patients in the two divisions was essentially the same, one significant difference did exist. The medical students comprising Division I performed daily cadaver dissections, whereas the student midwives of Division II did not. Rooting through old records, Semmelweis soon discovered some interesting facts that he thought might lend some insight into the cause of puerperal fever. Since each division after the separation in 1839 had to report its own mortality statistics, it allowed Semmelweis to see that it was the medical students in Division I that experienced mortality rates consistently higher than the student midwives of Division II.

He further discovered, as his Table I illustrates, that this difference was not a one-time event. During the six-year epoch from 1841 to 1846, Division I experienced infection rates consistently two to three times greater than those in the midwives' Division II—one of the first important truths he uncovered. The heightened danger of being admitted to Division I, rather than Division II, was even well known to the public. As Semmelweis described it: "The patients really do fear the first clinic. Frequently one must witness moving

One of sixty-four tables resulting from Semmelweis's research. This table demonstrates that, over a five-year epoch, mortality rates in Division I (9.92 percent) were nearly triple the 3.38 percent experienced in Division II.

Physicians, Division I					Midwives, Division II		
Year	Births	Deaths	%		Births	Deaths	%
1841	3036	237	7.8		2442	86	3.5
1842	3287	518	15.8		2659	202	7.5
1843	3060	274	8.9		2739	169	6.2
1844	3157	260	8.2		2956	68	2.3
1845	3492	241	6.9		3241	66	2.0
1846	4010	459	11.4		3754	105	2.7
TOTAL	20,042	1,989	9.92		17,791	696	3.9

scenes in which patients, kneeling and wringing their hands, beg to be released in order to seek admission to the second clinic. Such patients have usually been admitted because they are ignorant of the reputation of the first clinic, but they soon become suspicious because of the large number of doctors present."[12]

He surmised that this difference in mortality rates between the two groups must hold an important clue to the cause of puerperal fever.

Semmelweis extracted additional facts that he compiled into more graphs contrasting infection rates and deaths versus parity (first versus multiple deliveries), length of labor, month of delivery, premature births, or precipitous births before and after splitting the ward into two divisions, and so on. From this effort, he created six-ty-four tables graphically contrasting and illustrating any and all variables that might possibly be connected to puerperal infections and to mortality. Some facts that he had already sensed clinically he could now confirm with statistics. Multiparous women, those delivering for at least the second time, with their shorter labors and more frequent precipitous births, represented a decidedly lower risk when compared to the primiparous—those women delivering for the first time. Being primiparous with its prolonged labor, multiple pelvic exams, and increased chance of genital injury, represented a high-risk condition. In fact, if labor lasted over twenty-four hours, chances of contracting puerperal infection were virtually 100 percent. From his experience with the disease, Semmelweis also knew that, if the mother fell into a special risk category, such as being primiparous, her newborn shared that elevated risk with her.[13]

Statistics also confirmed another clinical observation: "street-births," that is, women who delivered at home or on the street prior to being admitted to the maternity ward, also represented a low-risk condition. They rarely became infected. Streetbirth mothers had a different hospital experience compared to the average patient. They required no trip to the labor room, and few if any internal exams, since they had already delivered. And their hospital stays after delivery were generally shorter. Interestingly, mortality rates in this low-risk group also did not differ appreciably between the two divisions. Exactly what factors protected this group from the mysterious infectious forces endemic to Division I remained a mystery. During the course of his research, Semmelweis would, on occasion, point out conundrums such as this to Professor Klein. From Klein's cool reception, it soon became obvious that the professor shared neither his assistant's enthusiasm nor his curiosity for the mystery. In fact, at a later date, after their relationship had further deteriorated, Klein, in full denial of the research, barred his assistant from gaining any further access to those records.[14]

Another enigma comparable to streetbirths involved women who delivered prematurely. Although subjected to the same general ward environment as the regular parturients, women experiencing premature births had rapid, generally complication-free deliveries that required few, if any, internal examinations. It was highly unlikely for this group of women to fall victim to puerperal fever—another unexplainable phenomenon.[15] It became obvious to Semmelweis that "streetbirths" and mothers of premature infants represented two low-risk groups. Each had mortality rates around 0.5 percent, or one in two hundred births, rates roughly comparable to women who delivered at home.[16] At this time, Semmelweis could do little more than duly note and store such facts in the back of his mind.

As these facts rose to the surface during his research, Semmelweis came to one conclusion: certain infectious factors were in play that pointed to puerperal fever, especially in Division I, being an endemic disease. In other words, puerperal fever existed within the ward, at some level, on a near-continual basis. The rate may fluctuate from time to time, but the disease was ever-present. Other aspects of the birth process in the Vienna Hospital, too numerous to list, would ultimately provide Semmelweis with detailed knowledge not only about mortality and patterns of propagation, but also other minor insights into puerperal fever that were unavailable to others. Semmelweis became locally known for the sixty-four tables that he generated from his research. When it came to informal discussions or argumentation with colleagues, being forearmed with such knowledge gave him a high level of confidence. How could adversaries level any sort of effective argument against someone who had such command of information? As he assembled facts, accepting some while rejecting others, getting a more informed grasp of how puerperal fever developed, his new insights sometimes allowed tentative answers to enigmas that left the average accoucheur scratching his head.[17] Although he could not yet articulate step-by-step how infection became established within the body, he had begun to question the wisdom of performing deliveries immediately after having performed cadaveric dissections.

As Semmelweis's departmental research progressed closer to his own era of assistantship, the mid-1840s, he found that the maternity service was delivering between three and four thousand women per year, or approximately ten deliveries per day. Mortality rates typically exceeded 6 percent. Of course, Professor Klein and his ilk still blithely attributed such high death rates to the *Genius epidemicus*. Although Semmelweis, with his diligent New School approach to the problem, remained well ahead of his contemporaries in his search for answers, he was still unable to offer any effective counterargument to their archaic notions. Perhaps his one remaining task, critiquing all contemporary puerperal fever theories, just might yield that one critical insight that could prove transformative.

Puerperal Fever Theories

Semmelweis's research of the literature constituted his least formal effort. He gained some enlightenment from formal readings, but a significant amount he gleaned during both his time as a trainee and, later, as he assumed his position as obstetrical assistant. Here, he had ample opportunity to utilize his prior exposure to formal logic as he examined the various theories. Although Semmelweis entered his assistantship with an unusual level of knowledge, already equipped with certain clinical impressions, he was astute enough to know that, when it came to formulating any new theories regarding the cause of puerperal fever, intuition, insights, and opinions gained through clinical experience alone were not sufficient. It would take a more ritualized process of examining the many existing theories, since none, so far, had proved satisfying to him.

Epidemic Causes

With the sheer numbers of European physicians still adhering to Sydenham's *Genius epidemicus* ideas of causation, it remained the dominant theory even as Semmelweis gained his medical degree. Physicians typically believed that disease resulted from multifactorial causes. Cosmic, atmospheric, or telluric forces, although of prime importance, could not be the sole cause in precipitating disease. It required at least one of a long supplemental list of predisposing factors including poor nutrition, chills, feelings of guilt (pregnancy out of wedlock), depression, even wearing too tight a petticoat, to actually make a disease blossom forth. Many felt that wounded modesty, epitomized by expectant women having to submit to that dreaded internal exam by men—male accoucheurs invading the most private feminine domain of pregnancy—could itself be a major factor in precipitating cases of puerperal fever. Some perfect storm of *Genius* forces, interacting with the expectant woman, predisposed through one or several of the above physical or psychic factors, caused the mysterious transformation from health to disease. No wonder the physicians' sense of complacency and fatalism. How could anyone prevent or combat a disease that was not only beyond one's control, but even beyond his comprehension? The very term *"Genius"* was an open declaration of ignorance.

According to the dominant doctrine, puerperal fever was a disease that existed on a minimal but continual baseline "sporadic," or endemic, level. Superimposed upon this endemic state were epidemic bursts, which occurred consequent to the influence of *Genius epidemicus*. Even under the most ideal of circumstances, its incidence could never be much lower than 1 percent among pregnant women. That was the "ideal" level of endemicity towards which a practitioner should strive. Of course, Semmelweis rejected the *Genius* theory. First, if *G. epidemicus* were in force, Divisions I and II should be equally affected. Otherwise one would have to postulate that atmospheric influences, considered so important to the epidemic theory, materialized and vanished every twenty-four hours in perfect coordination with the admission schedules of the two divisions. Also, if epidemic influences were so powerful, a much larger geographic area should be involved, not just the limited borders of one hospital ward. It was an incontrovertible fact that the disease could be raging on one hospital ward and yet not a single case exist in the adjacent ward, or even within the city. Semmelweis soon became contemptuous enough of the illogic of this theory that, in later arguments with colleagues, he would often reveal his ongoing frustration by referring derisively to adherents of this theory as "epidemicists."

Secondly, Semmelweis became convinced that the four seasons had no significant effect on the disease. It was true that, in general, the number of cases of childbed fever increased slightly in the winter months and decreased in the summertime, but he could easily explain that away by looking at student activity. In the summer, they preferred to study outside enjoying the green grass and blue skies, while in the winter they escaped the cold by spending the major part of their time dissecting in the morgue. Thirdly, a simple fact of puerperal fever kept surfacing, one that he could not ignore. Puerperal infection invariably occurred in association with trauma to some part of the birth canal. He could think of no other sort of epidemic disease that bore such a critical relationship to trauma.[1]

Cosmic-Atmospheric-Telluric Forces

Tied in closely with the *Genius* doctrine was the popular "cosmic-atmospheric-telluric" theory. In essence, this theory was little more than a recent, broad-based iteration of Sydenham's two types of *Genius*—the *epidemicus* and *dyscrasis*. It dealt with any cause originating in the cosmos, the atmosphere, or the earth. Semmelweis, with his diligent reading and daily experience with patients, had already seen enough of this theory to view it as invalid. He could discard it employing the same lines of reasoning as he had for the *G. epidemicus* theory. If childbed fever were an epidemic disease, subject to temperature, barometric pressure, and wind direction, why then did its geographic spread not mirror the patterns of weather and the like? Should not the atmospheric factors rain down equally on all geographic areas subjected to those factors? Practitioners who employed this theory could not explain how cases occurred in a single row of beds or in alternate rows. Why would one discrete part of a ward become infected when the adjacent ward, the general hospital, and the town itself, all subject to the same weather influences, remain disease-free? If one applied this same logic to Divisions I and II, with each division admitting on alternate days, the theory becomes even more absurd. Did atmospheric conditions vary every twenty-four hours in perfect coordination with the admitting schedule of each maternity ward? Both divisions were subjected to the same atmospheric conditions. If such diseased areas were the result of atmospheric conditions, they should all be affected equally. And, clearly, they were not.

As Semmelweis pondered many other purported causes of puerperal fever, he came to view them as equally absurd. If wounded modesty were a factor, as many claimed, how was it that women in the higher classes, whether delivering at home or in private clinics, did not experience the higher rates of infection seen on charity wards? They were commonly attended by men. Did they not suffer the same degree of wounded modesty as the women in Division I? The shame of the unmarried, "fallen" women occupying Vienna's wards was also considered an important factor in causing puerperal fever. Since each division drew from the same human reservoir, then rates in Divisions I and II should be equal. Using his *per exclusionem* method, Semmelweis therefore had to discard shame as a force in causation. He could just as easily exclude another popular factor as a sole cause of puerperal infection—lack of ventilation. Since all factors of cross-ventilation, such as ward design, height and numbers of windows, and the like, were virtually identical in the two divisions, infections and deaths should be the same in Divisions I and II. Yet, that clearly was not the case. The same logic could be applied to other conditions, such as chilling and poor diet, since such variables did not differ appreciably between patient populations on the two wards.[2]

Miasmatic Causes

Another idea closely related to the epidemic, contagionist, and cosmic-atmospheric-telluric theories was one concerning "vitiated" (contaminated) or "miasmatic" air. Such air contained "zymotic" particles, that is, particles that were both invisible and infectious. It was a well-known fact that diseases were much more prevalent in any area in which overcrowding and general filth existed. Scientists postulated that particles, whether organic or inorganic, thrived in this foul or miasmatic air. When such particles, or "zymes," lit upon some unlucky individual, a zymotic disease ensued—a view not too unlike our modern-day concept of infectious diseases, except this view was born of pure speculation. Most physicians considered it unwise to live anywhere near swamps, sloughs, or open sewers. One might be able to avoid zymotic contact, say from a sewer, when active during the day, but as nighttime ensued, it was a different story. As fluids evaporated during the heat of day, zymotic particles could become suspended in the air, floating freely for hours. Then with the arrival of morning, these same airborne sewer particles might be blown over a sleeping individual just as the temperature changed, inducing a condensation—the morning dew. Those same particles then landed on some unsuspecting individual, primed for a zymotic or miasmatic disease. Any prudent physician subscribing to this theory would advise his expectant patient to move away from such noxious sources not just during her pregnancy, but for several weeks after her delivery.

This miasmatic view became further entrenched in physicians' minds after some memorable epidemics of puerperal fever. In 1664, the most notable one occurred at the Hotel Dieu in Paris. When obstetricians discovered abscesses consistently in the autopsies of puerperal fever victims, they connected the high infection rate to the surgical ward's proximate location underneath the maternity wing. They immediately concluded that: "Coarse and infectious vapors, which arose from the wounds and ulcers of the wounded bodies, created a mass of impure and malignant air. The air perpetually rose upward and was inhaled day and night by the newly delivered women. The women fell into a bloody flux that ended only with their death."[3]

With subsequent epidemics in other large European hospitals, each occurring under similar circumstances, obstetricians on the Continent looked back on these preceding epidemics as proof that malignant, miasmatic air was the cause. Dirty air was omnipresent. It had to be intimately connected to disease causation. As such ideas grew more deeply embedded, the more difficult it became for physicians to discard them when confronted by competing theories.

Miscellaneous Theories

Multiple other lesser-known theories existed, with fewer adherents. The theory of "milk metastasis" arose as a result of physicians attempting to connect two common observations: milk production commonly diminished in the presence of puerperal fever just as yellow-white exudates consistently appeared in the bodily cavities. Since physiology hardly existed as a scientific discipline in the early nineteenth century, physicians had little idea how the body actually functioned. Some adherents of this theory believed milk production continued but in some way it metastasized to the abdominal and chest cavities. They were convinced that the yellow-white exudates were nothing but putrefied milk, mysteriously curdled, as it was being deposited in the bodily cavities.[4] Apparently no one had ever placed a sample of the exudate on a slide for examination under a microscope. Such a theory was easy for Semmelweis to discard.

Some theorists considered the intestines, along with the gravid uterus, to be intimately intertwined in the production of puerperal fever. They postulated that, late in pregnancy as the uterus enlarged, an obstruction of flow occurred within the intestines. Treatment was obvious—purgatives and multiple enemas. Obstetrician John Leake was so impressed with the foul odor of peritonitis noted at autopsy that he mistakenly believed the process originated from within the intestines. Consequently, he preferred the name "putrid flatus," rather than puerperal fever. Some, like Manchester surgeon Charles White, believed that childbed fever resulted from putrid bowel matter that, in some inscrutable way, contaminated the uterus. He envisioned a vicious circle of infection beginning with vitiated or "miasmatic" air resulting from generally poor ventilation, closed windows, overcrowding, and dirty linens. His solution? Get rid of all soiled items such as sheets and bed clothes, encourage cross ventilation, avoid warm atmospheres by prohibiting fires, and so on.[5] Although White's advocacy for cleanliness made sense, Semmelweis recognized the absurdity of White's theory, as well as some others that could be eliminated outright.

The theory of fibrin enjoyed some popularity. Fibrin, that clotting constituent within blood, was also considered a prominent factor in the etiology of many inflammatory diseases, including puerperal fever. This theory originated after physicians noted that patients who died with overwhelming inflammation had, at autopsy, prominent deposits of fibrin throughout their abdominal and chest organs, much like Semmelweis would have noted in the prominent exudates of his puerperal fever victims. Those scientists, generally adherents of humoralism, postulated that the fibrin content increased in the blood in response to whatever unknown stimulus it was that caused a particular disease. In the case of puerperal fever, it was fibrin within the mother's blood that led to the degeneration or crasis. Rokitansky, despite his generally pioneering and modern views, believed in the fibrinous theory as the cause of puerperal fever, a view he would hold until the latter 1840s.

Gordon of Aberdeen

Near the turn of the eighteenth century, one important theory on puerperal fever arose in Scotland, through the efforts of retired naval surgeon Alexander Gordon. At the time that Semmelweis was conducting his own research, he was probably unaware of Gordon's work from fifty years earlier, given the undeveloped state of medical journalism, limitations of long distance travel, and the different languages between the two countries. Semmelweis would, however, be confronted with Gordon's work in the years after he had announced his own theory. He was aware that the British had noted a general association between puerperal fever and erysipelas, a well-known, highly contagious disease of the skin. Since the British had the lowest rates of puerperal infection in the Western world, their assertions had to be taken seriously. They based their contagionist views primarily upon the work of two different men, the first of whom was Gordon, a naval surgeon. Upon retiring from the navy, Gordon engaged in a practice in Aberdeen, where he was immediately confronted with a withering epidemic of childbed fever. Gordon responded by conducting one of the earliest high quality epidemiologic studies of childbirth ever, before the modern era. He discovered a close correlation between puerperal fever and cases of erysipelas. With its bright scarlet color and raised, discrete margins, one could diagnose erysipelas from ten feet away. In fact, with its sharp edges, one might mistake it, at first glance, for a tattoo.

Gordon made some important discoveries by actually tracing the treatment itineraries of certain village physicians as they attended deliveries or cared for patients with erysipelas. Even though erysipelas was considered to be a contagious disease, most physicians exercised no special precautions after caring for a patient with the disease. It was also not at all unusual to find both physicians and midwives, after having treated patients afflicted with erysipelas in one setting, to proceed directly to attend women in labor. Practitioners neither washed their hands nor changed their clothes in between these two tasks. As Gordon traced the movements of Aberdeen midwives, he discovered that they left a consistent and traceable number of puerperal fever victims in their wake. With such nonchalance, if not blind ignorance of causation, an epidemic inevi-

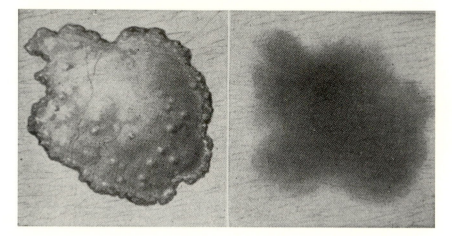

Figure 16. The lesion of erysipelas on the left, compared to the more nonspecific inflammation of the deeper tissues on the right. Note that erysipelas is
raised, has blisters on its surface, and has margins so discrete that it could
be mistaken for a tattoo. The lesion on the right appears more cloud-like and
exhibits less distinct borders. Taken from *New People's Physician*, Vol. 5 (New
York: William H. Wise and Company, 1942): 1,348.

tably ensued, beginning in December 1789. Despite peaking in 1790,
it persisted until the spring of 1792.[6] Gordon was so convinced of
the association of the two diseases that he used the term, "puerperal
erysipelas" instead of puerperal fever.[7] Excited about his discovery,
he enthusiastically published his results in 1795, proclaiming, "I
have unquestionable proof . . . [it] seized such women only, as were
visited, or delivered, by a practitioner, or taken care of by a nurse,
who had previously attended patients affected by the disease."[8]
When Gordon naively included the names of the offending practitioners in his treatise, he faced such wrath from those he had named
that he was forced to terminate his research. He retreated back to
less contentious waters by rejoining the Navy. Let those Aberdeen
practitioners solve their own problems.

James Simpson

The second British contagionist was Edinburgh professor James
Simpson, Queen Victoria's own accoucheur. Like Gordon, he had
not only been aware of a longstanding association between puer-

peral fever and erysipelas, he also knew that this highly infectious disease ran rampant on general medical and surgical wards. He believed that it was the fingers of medical attendants that, however innocently, implanted *"materies morbi"* into the "dilated and abraded living membrane of the maternal passages." Semmelweis, as he carried out his research before 1847, was unaware of Simpson's work. Simpson was similarly unaware of Semmelweis when, in 1850, approximately four years after Semmelweis, he described in an essay the clinical courses and the full spectrum of manifestations of such erysipelas-related infections.[9] The most common variant of this skin infection was impetigo, a disease of the upper-most layer of the skin. Although serious, it was generally not life-threatening, often resolving spontaneously. Erysipelas, which involved mainly the middle layer of skin, was clearly the most dangerous of the common group.

But the most aggressive and terrifying form of these skin diseases, gangrenous erysipelas (necrotizing fasciitis in modern parlance), involved the tissues immediately beneath the skin rather than the dermis itself. The virulence of this disease is attributable to the bacterial release of an enzyme that literally dissolves all surrounding tissues, eating away within a matter of hours muscles, fat, tendons and ligaments, or any other tissue residing in the area. In the nineteenth century, sepsis from gangrenous erysipelas was terrifying, brief, and invariably fatal.[10]

Typical lesions of erysipelas were easy to spot. The patient first experienced scarlet streaks somewhere on the trunk or extremities—cutaneous manifestations of the inflammation lying deeper within the blood and lymphatic vessels. Along with malaise and fever, these red streaks in the skin were the premonitory signs of puerperal fever. In the 1840s, these infections were sufficiently commonplace that Semmelweis and his contemporaries, even though they did not understand the reason behind such lesions, could readily foresee the impending scenario: scarlet streaks coalescing into broader islands of reddened tissues, which then turn blue-black. As the vessels become completely obstructed by inflammation, death of the surrounding tissues inevitably occurred. Next, in the more serious cases, came the blood crasis (septicemia), with its teeth-rattling rigors, stupor, and confusion, as some sort of "toxin" entered the circulation, affecting all organs, all tissues of the body. Death followed soon after. It would not be until 1883 that German surgeon Friedrich Fehleinsen cultured streptococcus from an erysipelas wound, establishing its true etiological agent.[11] Researchers later discovered that streptococcus was the common bacterial cause of all three skin diseases.

Early in Semmelweis's quest he concluded that the contagionist theory, as conceived by Gordon and later Simpson, and enthusiastically received by the British, was not a tenable explanation of causation. While they achieved low rates of infection by following some general rules of behavior, their contagionist theory was not a stepwise elucidation of a particular biologic process. They had merely relied upon some empiric observations in building their program of prophylaxis. Semmelweis's critical review of all relevant puerperal fever theories existing in the 1840s had to have given him further perspective about what causation was and was not. While the disease may be communicable, it was not infectious in the sense that one expectant woman sharing close quarters with another could easily pass the disease on to her neighbor, as happened with cholera or smallpox, for example.

Oliver Wendell Holmes

One American physician, Oliver Wendell Holmes, although having no direct clinical or research experience in obstetrics, came very close to solving the enigma of puerperal fever by merely conducting a meta-analysis, an extensive review of much of the world's literature on the disease. In his reading, he observed that whenever practitioners treated a variety of patients suffering from various inflammatory conditions, such as gangrene, peritonitis, as well as erysipelas, prior to attending women in labor, those parturients suffered a disproportionate number of deaths consequent to puerperal fever. "The conclusion is irresistible that a most fearful morbid poison is often generated in the course of this disease [puerperal fever]. Whether or not it is *sui generis*, confined to this disease, or produced in some others, as for instance erysipelas, I need not stop to inquire."[12] Holmes had merely noted that diseases that today would be called "infectious," were associated with unusually high rates of puerperal infection. In 1843, he published his conclusions in an essay, "The Contagiousness of Puerperal Fever." It is doubtful that Semmelweis was aware of Holmes's work, which preceded his own by a mere four years. Holmes did not pretend to have an explanation as to the manner in which the disease was propagated; he merely pointed out the undeniable association between the two diseases. Holmes suggested some rules of conduct for practitioners. If caring for expectant women, do not perform autopsies. If treating patients with erysipelas, wait twenty-four hours and change clothing completely before attending to any woman in labor. Holmes went so far as to state that he considered it a criminal act to attend to a woman in labor without observing the simple precautions that he had outlined. But Holmes's article, just like Gordon's four decades earlier, caused an explosion of hostile responses from the ranks of obstetricians. Charles Meigs, the prominent Philadelphia professor, the same Meigs who had praised Sydenham for his humoralist theories, publicly rebuked Holmes for his "sophomoric" musings. He suggested that the young Holmes should stick to his own field of anatomy. Holmes did just that by later becoming professor of anatomy at Harvard Medical School. It was just too difficult for Meigs and most other obstetricians to accept the idea that a physician could actually be causing such large numbers of this dreaded disease: *How could I, having the best of intentions, possibly be guilty of causing such suffering and death?*

As the British began to fully appreciate the infectious nature of these diseases, erysipelas in particular, they established certain rules of behavior similar to Holmes's admonitions: after caring for a patient with erysipelas or puerperal fever, it is prudent to bathe and change clothing completely; if more than one case of puerperal fever occurs under your care, take several weeks off from your practice to allow whatever process is in play to dissipate. Borrowing from an old French agricultural practice of decontamination, English obstetricians began the pragmatic use of chloride of lime as a general cleanser. Even though they did not understand the rationale behind its use, they hoped it would prevent the disease. The practice proved valid. Despite occasional sporadic epidemics, the British enjoyed low levels of puerperal fever merely by the using the chloride regimen and following the above simple rules of conduct. European obstetricians, whether through ignorance or contempt for the British theory, exercised no such precautions.

Semmelweis's own views on the disease evolved into something close to the British, yet their theory was less than satisfying to him. The British considered puerperal fever to be a more contagious disease than did Semmelweis. He saw no evidence that it could be passed on from one patient to another as readily as say, cholera or smallpox might be. In other words, it was not a disease, *sui generis*—its own species of disease. And, as mentioned, the British had merely pointed out the association between the two diseases. Semmelweis needed to know what mechanism lay behind this contagion. Without that answer, neither he nor the British had a tenable and satisfying theory.

Autopsy Experience

Semmelweis's grim task of dissecting hundreds of puerperal fever victims over the past two years had paid significant dividends when it came to understanding the abnormal anatomy consequent to puerperal fever. The sober, monotonously consistent pathologic findings allowed him to, at least, make certain generalizations. The earliest signs of trouble, scarlet streaking in the soft tissues of the upper-inner thighs and external genitalia, indicated inflammatory changes in the surrounding vessels and lymphatics, a harbinger not only of tissue death (necrosis) but of worse to come. After observing the same unwavering findings in many consecutive autopsies, Semmelweis concluded that the uterus and its surrounding tissues near the pelvic floor, plus the external private parts, lay at the epicenter of inflammation. The uterus and those surrounding tissues appeared to be the anatomic site in which the disease process originated—the first of several anatomic constants.

Another constant, inescapable fact in patients dying of puerperal fever, was the great volumes of yellow-white exudates present in the major bodily cavities of all puerperal fever victims. From where did the exudates arise, and why did they appear? The full explanation for their presence would have to await two events. In 1858, the English surgeon Joseph Lister performed some pioneering microscopic studies viewing capillaries in the webbed feet of frogs. He discovered that as inflammation worsened, capillaries in the area became paralyzed and patulous, allowing the free escape of blood cells across the vessel walls. Thirty years later, in 1876, Julius Cohnheim demonstrated that pus, which was nothing more than millions of white blood cells and tissue detritus, arose in response to any strong inflammatory stimulus. Pus cells, normally constituents of circulating blood, escaped across the capillary walls to combat any toxins residing within the inflamed tissues. This was pus, but in the 1840s, that fact was not yet appreciated.[13] No wonder some practitioners believed the exudates to be curdled, fermented milk.

Even though Semmelweis was ignorant of what exudates were or how they formed, he accepted them as constants in patients dying of puerperal fever. The same questions that plagued him regarding exudates he could direct to another constant, as well. Abscesses, those randomly scattered aggregations of metastasized infectious material, whether microscopic or visible to the naked eye, were always identifiable within specific organs such as the liver, lungs, or heart. Wherever there was circulation within the body—which was everywhere—micro-abscesses could occur.

Regardless of whatever order these constants appeared, Semmelweis recognized yet a fourth one—the degenerative ferment that developed within the bloodstream. Whether one called the process a "crasis," a "ferment," a "dissolution," a "pyemia," or a "sepsis," each referred to the same physiological state. He knew that this abnormal state of the blood invariably occurred after the onset of peritonitis, and before the rapid deterioration that resulted in death. From his clinical experience alone, Semmelweis recognized this ferment of blood to be the invariable harbinger of death. Was it the common denominator behind all the other tissue changes seen in puerperal fever victims at autopsy?

As Semmelweis's departmental research brought him more into the present, the mid-1840s, and mortality rates continuously hovered between 6 and 10 percent, *Genius epidemicus* was still considered the common cause. Although Semmelweis continued making significant strides forward in his research, he was painfully aware that he could not yet claim to have arrived at any sort of definitive solution. His gains still provided no practical remedy for improving the unacceptable maternal infection rates. These were the facts of

puerperal fever as seen by Semmelweis around the time he concluded his two years in waiting, as he anxiously anticipated the beginning of his assistantship.

Assistantship

July 1846: Finally Semmelweis could step up to the position he had coveted for more than two years. He began his formal assistantship, arguably the best prepared and the most highly informed trainee ever entering his respective field of specialization at Vienna General Hospital. Yet, his assignment would last only four months.

Semmelweis faced an onerous workload, running this gargantuan department at the pleasure of his professor, Johann Klein. As the assistant, he was responsible for all patient care, teaching of medical students, maintaining all departmental records, performing all operations and deliveries within Division I, and assisting Klein with operations on the professor's private patients. The physical demands made patient care, by itself, more than a full time job. On one occasion Semmelweis performed thirty-four deliveries in the course of a single twenty-four-hour period.[1] Each morning, Semmelweis would conduct his working rounds, rounds designed mainly to resolve patient problems on the ward, with a full retinue of medical students in tow. Then there were the more formal rounds with Professor Klein every afternoon, a time devoted more to student instruction. On top of that heavy load, Semmelweis continued not only with his morning dissections in the morgue, but with all aspects of his research, as well. He kept his statistics up to date by continuing to compile infection and mortality rates. Such a workload gave him virtually no time for any sort of social life, no more waltzing the women in the dance halls, no more days off to simply reenergize. With no time to cultivate new friendships, let alone maintain old ones, the demands of his work rendered him virtually asocial.[2] In fact, he remained so dedicated, so determined to find the answer to the mystery of puerperal fever, that he took no vacations during his entire assistantship, save for one soon-to-be-mentioned respite.

As multiple biographers have noted, changes soon became evident in Semmelweis. "This gay, carefree young student of Vienna had developed into the most active and painstaking doctor in the hospital."[3] Despite his two years of study and autopsy experience, it took but little time after settling in before the stark reality of puerperal fever began to weigh on him psychologically. Shortly before he began his assistantship, mortality rates ran so high that the ministry convened a formal commission to study the problem. Commission members began interrogating all departmental faculty members hoping to come up with some causes and to render a solution. During one such interrogation of Klein, the professor told the committee that Vienna's high infection rates were attributable to "bad conditions" within the hospital walls, implying that miasmatic air was the ultimate cause. Upon hearing Klein's obvious misstatement, Semmelweis, who was standing nearby, rose immediately to contradict his professor, stating that many hospitals throughout Europe have walls more contaminated than those in Vienna, yet they do not experience the same magnitude of puerperal fever as that seen in Vienna. Miasmatic air could not be the common source.[4] Klein, instantly angered, could do little but bite his tongue, since members of the commission were still present. The incident, however, represented one of the first strikes against his new assistant. It took little time for Klein to develop a simmering dislike for the tactless, overly forthright young assistant who, had he ever heard the unspoken rule concerning deference to persons in authority, never bothered to follow it. No doubt Semmelweis, armed with his new research, entered his assistantship supremely confidant, feeling little need to measure his words whatever the circumstance. He knew more about the great scourge of puerperal infection than those who were instructing him. Such actions and attitudes noted by superiors during the course of his training eventually earned him the title of "ungovernable."[5] Thus, the tone of Semmelweis's assistantship at Vienna General Hospital was set.

As Semmelweis labored on, seeing the depressingly high numbers of infections and deaths in Division I, a lassitude as insidious as the morning fog set in. Daily, he saw young women in the terminal throes of puerperal fever, with abdominal pain more excruciating than labor itself. He became haunted by their screams piercing the night air. Dealing with a disease that nobody really understood, that had no effective treatment, reduced his own role as caregiver to that of feckless observer. Add to that his autopsy experience, dealing with dead bodies ravaged by pyemia. With no effective way to gain any respite, it required but a few months for his angst to become inescapable.

As he continued collecting departmental statistics, even contrasting the mortality rates in the two divisions gave him a heightened sense of guilt. His own Division I had rates consistently around 6 percent, while Division II was a more respectable 2 percent.[6] Why the difference? What was going on in Division I? Semmelweis became ever more dispirited, a mere observer forced to confront an insurmountable problem.

As he struggled on, Semmelweis began to suspect that the internal exams performed by staff and students immediately after dissecting cadavers must, in some way, be connected to the high incidence of puerperal fever in Division I. Still, as he weighed various potential etiologies, the ultimate cause of the disease evaded him. Why could he not make the connection? As he later recounted, "I couldn't discover in the hitherto prevailing principles underlying the etiology of puerperal fever the actual existence of the alleged etiologic factors in the many hundreds of cases which I saw treated in vain."[7] Heavy hearted over his own ineffectiveness and that of medicine in general, his melancholy deepened. "A feeling of discouragement had taken possession of me . . . really and truly I would have preferred to die," he lamented. "The puerperal disease remains a mystery, only the number of the dead is a palpable fact."[8] Even Marko noted the torment and changes already suggestive of obsession in his roommate, wrought by his own fecklessness. He explained, "I had the chance of seeing him [Semmelweis], both in the hospital and at home—his watchful restlessness, his eagerness to examine people and conditions, his prying eyes trying to penetrate into the murderous disease, his zest to discover its cause."[9] Although neither yet admitted it overtly, Semmelweis was in the early stages of his first significant bout with depression.

Then two unexpected events added further to Semmelweis's torment. Later in 1846, his beloved father died without warning, a loss the devoted son would not soon overcome. Then, another major blow: on October 20, 1846, with no warning whatsoever, Klein relieved Semmelweis of his assistantship, after only four months of training. Klein used the excuse that Semmelweis's immediate predecessor in Division I, Gustave Breit, wished to return to his old position. Suddenly Semmelweis was faced with another period of forced inactivity, a hiatus that would last five months.[10]

Venice

Semmelweis was too dispirited to recognize his opportunity immediately, but just being separated from his depressive environment would turn into his good fortune. After spending time contemplating what he might do with his unwanted spare time, he decided to follow the path of the iconic Johann Boer by visiting obstetricians in the United Kingdom. He began to study English in anticipation of traveling first to Dublin, where he hoped to gain insights by better learning the Irish approach to puerperal fever. But Marko, sensing his friend's level of despondency, suggested a more practical solution—a purely frivolous trip to Venice. No doubt, a drastic change of scene would be beneficial for him—an escape from his weighty obsession. As Semmelweis reminisced later, he agreed to the trip to "refresh his depressed spirits very much tried by the events in the clinic."[11] Those three weeks that he, Marko, and another friend spent touring the Venetian treasure houses of art did seem the ideal prescription. He was moved enough to later describe Venice as "an enchanted city, its art works beyond compare."[12] Semmelweis's spirits were much lifted as the trip concluded. While having no expectations about returning to work in Division I, he did feel a resurgence of his old enthusiasm to continue his pursuit of puerperal fever.

As the trio returned to Vienna, Semmelweis received two surprise announcements. First, Breit's tenure as Division I assistant had proved extraordinarily brief. Almost as soon as he had begun work, he was offered the professorship in Tubingen. He took no time at all to accept the post. Suddenly the way for Semmelweis was clear again. On March 20, 1847, he resumed his old job filled with resurgent vigor. If he stopped to consider the wisdom of placing himself once again in such a depressive atmosphere under the hostile Klein, after barely recovering from his first bout of acute depression, it was not apparent. The stage was set for Semmelweis's second assistantship, an era that would evolve, both for Semmelweis and the entire medical faculty, into one of the most memorable and contentious of all eras at Vienna General Hospital.[13]

Enlightenment

Semmelweis's second surprise greeted him soon after his return from Venice, when he visited the Old Rifle Factory to organize his resumption of autopsy duties. As Semmelweis entered, he was immediately puzzled by the expectant look given him by the technician in charge. Had he heard the news about Kolletschka? When Semmelweis replied in the negative, he was stunned by the technician's revelations. His friend, the popular professor of forensics had died on March 13, just one week before Semmelweis's return. How could it be? Kolletschka was only forty-four and in good health a mere three weeks ago. As Semmelweis listened in stunned silence, the technician related how, during a forensic dissection, a medical student had accidently cut one of Kolletschka's index fingers with an autopsy knife. The cut was small. Initially, there seemed no cause for concern. But soon Kolletschka began feeling ill with fever and general malaise. Then came the red streaks coursing up his arm, typical of one suffering from inflammation of the lymphatic and blood vessels (lymphangitis and vasculitis). Then, sadly, Kolletschka deteriorated rapidly, with high fever and confusion progressing to coma. As Semmelweis heard how fulminating Kolletschka's terminal event had been, he could only conclude that his friend had died from sepsis.

Kolletschka's autopsy was performed in the same morgue in which he had himself spent so many hours working. Semmelweis, after examining a copy of the pathologist's report, was as intrigued as he was horrified and saddened. Kolletschka exhibited extensive tissue death in his arm due to occlusion of the vessels and lymphatics. Just as startling, his abdominal and chest cavities and the sac around his heart were filled with milky-white exudates, diagnostic of peritonitis, pleuritis, and pericarditis. He had meningitis, as well, marked by the presence of exudates throughout his cerebrospinal fluid. Additionally, the pathologist noted abscesses, scattered at random, throughout his major organs. The most dramatic of all findings was a large abscess residing within his left eye socket causing gross displacement of the globe. Semmelweis's suspicions were confirmed. Kolletschka had died of sepsis.

Enlightenment

As Semmelweis related years later, "Day and night this picture of Kolletschka's disease pursued me and with ever increasing determination, I was obliged to acknowledge the identity of the disease, from which Kolletschka died, with that disease of which I saw so many puerperae die."[1] A friend's unexpected death might merely be passed over by ordinary associates as an extremely unfortunate event. But Semmelweis, as he confronted this shocking incident, had an advantage over his contemporaries. His mind was preconditioned, his pump primed, with all of the facts he had gleaned through his years of research. Unlike the practitioner languishing in *Genius* theory, insight came to Semmelweis as an explosive revelation. Both groups of patients had succumbed to a miliary process. The signs and symptoms of Kolletschka's rapid decline and death were identical to the monotonously constant clinical pictures of those hundreds of puerperal fever victims that Semmelweis had himself autopsied over the years. They too, had findings of vasculitis, peritonitis, pleuritis, meningitis, plus exudates in their bodily cavities and abscesses scattered at random throughout their internal organs. Obviously Kolletschka had no genital wound, but otherwise their diseases were identical. The source of Kolletschka's illness and demise was his finger laceration by a knife contaminated with some sort of toxic particles residing within the cadaver. These particles then gained entrance directly into his bloodstream via the laceration, causing sepsis followed by that sad infectious cascade leading to his death, a death that followed the identical steps by which all the new mothers passed on. As Semmelweis saw it, both Kolletschka and those many victims of puerperal fever had one element in common. The soft-tissue wounds of each group, regardless of location, had to have been contaminated by toxic cadaveric particles.

Once Semmelweis recognized the commonality of these diseases, connected via the development of sepsis, further revelations flooded in. Cadaveric contamination of soft-tissue wounds would explain why patients in Division II did not suffer the same high rates of infection as in Division I. Student midwives did not dissect cadavers. Therefore, they did not contaminate the genital tract when they performed their internal exams. The same could even be said for the low rates of infection for practitioners in the city. They did not dissect cadavers and therefore did not carry contaminants to their patients.

Gravid women in the hospital, on the other hand, were examined by physicians and medical students, usually fresh from the dissecting room, with bare hands contaminated by the stink of cadaveric material. Instead of a laceration like Kolletschka, these same particles were brought into contact with the wounded birth canals of the laboring women via the examining physician's hands. The one common element causing death in both Kolletschka and the new mothers was wounds contaminated by cadaveric particles. They merely had wounds in different parts of their bodies. Once the toxic material penetrated the injured tissues of the wound, it gained access into the patient's bloodstream, setting up that same final common pathway to death.[2] It was the existence of the wound, not its location, that was the critical element.

Even in those newborns that died alongside their infected mothers, the autopsy findings were the same, absent the genital component. Since the mothers shared the same circulation with their infants, the mothers transferred the contaminant, some type of toxic cadaveric particles, directly to their offspring via the umbilical cord. It could occur either immediately before or during the birthing process. That was the one element common to the groups of expectant women, their newborns, and the groups of surgeons and pathologists who were accidently cut during the course of their work. Kolletschka was a prime example of the latter group. After being contaminated via different routes, their bedside manifestations of the disease, regardless of their group or site of wound, were superimposable as they progressed on to death from a condition common to both—pyemia. Suddenly, it all seemed so clear![3]

As Semmelweis contemplated the ramifications of his discovery, he was humbled as he considered the consequences of his own prior behavior. How many thousands of times had he himself proceeded directly from the morgue to the maternity ward to examine expectant women, most of whom were in labor? Though his mistakes were committed in innocent ignorance, Semmelweis realized the depth of his own guilt in causing epidemics of puerperal fever and offered the public the first of two *mea culpas*: "My conscience tells me that I must reprove myself, as God only knows the number of those who have died as a result of my activity. Few of the obstetricians have had more dealings with cadavers than myself . . . However painful and distressing this fact is, there would be no sense in denying it. No, there is one remedy only: to publish the truth to all those who are concerned."[4]

Shortly after making his great inductive leap concerning the cause of puerperal fever, he made another important decision regarding its prevention. If his hypothesis concerning the entrance of cadaveric particles into the vascular system by merely coming into contact with genital wounds was correct, then why not destroy those same particles with some sort of chemical? He was already aware that several European cities deodorized their sewage systems using chloride of lime. Knowing nothing about bacteria, Semmelweis merely equated the putrid stench remaining on the anatomist's hands after his perfunctory soapy wash with the persistence of cadaveric matter. If the aroma persisted after a wash, then the contaminant was still present. Conversely: get rid of the odor with chloride of lime, and the toxic matter should be gone. With that rationale, Semmelweis decided that all personnel, including custodians, nurses, students, and faculty, must wash in chloride of lime, including using a brush underneath the fingernails, until the putrefactive odor was completely gone.

In early May 1847, Semmelweis met with Professor Klein to explain his new theory and his program for prophylaxis. "Puerperal fever is caused by cadaveric particles adhering to the hands of the physician who examines the childbed patients," he explained, "thus it is of utmost importance that he should clean his hands properly before a visit, for which purpose I advise the chlorine solution."[5] Semmelweis then outlined, in greater detail, his proposed regimen of washing the hands and brushing underneath the fingernails with the chloride solution, not superficially, but diligently until all cadaveric odor is gone. He recommended to Klein that all personnel wash in this manner, not only as they enter the ward prior to any patient contact, but also before all operations. Since the chances of contamination were less once a student was on the ward and had already gone through the chloride regimen once, a simple washing with soap and water in between subsequent patient exams should be sufficient.

Surprisingly, Klein, who had displayed no interest in Semmelweis's research whatsoever, went along with the plan without fully understanding its rationale. When medical students, nurses, and midwives considered the level of inconvenience such a regimen would entail, they protested loudly, but with Klein's imprimatur, the program went into effect in mid-May 1847. Amazingly, Klein himself even participated in the washings in full compliance with Semmelweis's new rules.

Once Klein had issued the chloride of lime edict, student resistance faded, and all personnel complied fully. It required less than four weeks of new mortality statistics for Semmelweis to realize that something profound was afoot: April, 18.3 percent; May, 12.2 percent; June, 2.4 percent. As he compiled the statistics for August, he was thrilled to discover that not one infection had occurred during the entire month.

But Klein appeared unmoved by the dramatic decrease in mortality rates. Adolf Kussmaul, who had worked under Semmelweis during this period of illumination, related that at no time did Klein display any interest whatsoever in the work of his young assistant. How could he remain apathetic and agnostic given Semmelweis's early results? Sadly, Klein would remain "a stumbling block, not so much because he wanted to oppose him, but for sheer lack of understanding." It became obvious to Semmelweis. Klein could never be counted on for any help.[6]

But before Semmelweis could get too excited with his early success, more problems arose. In October 1847, an expectant woman suffering from a chronically infected, draining carcinoma of the cervix was admitted to Division I. Her bed was situated such that it was the first one Semmelweis and students encountered as they began their rounds. Per their new routine, all doctors scrubbed in the chlorine bowl before examining patients, then all proceeded first to the patient in bed one, at this time the patient with cancer. After examining her, they proceeded consecutively to the other patients in the same row of beds, only washing with soap and water in between each patient. Within days, disaster struck. Eleven out of twelve patients in that row of beds died of puerperal fever, causing Semmelweis great consternation. The events surrounding this woman's infection shook the very foundation of his entire theory as to how puerperal fever is propagated. Beginning a serious reassessment of his theory, he pondered, *"Could the miasmatists have a point after all? Was some type of specific zyme or miasm hanging over small, discrete areas of the ward?"*

As Semmelweis continued struggling, trying to make sense of this disaster, a second problem arose in November, only one month later. On this occasion, a gravid woman with chronic osteomyelitis of her knee, draining "ichorous material," was admitted to the maternity wing. Again, a geographic cluster of deaths occurred surrounding this woman and her bed. As Semmelweis contemplated these new facts, trying to integrate them into his new heuristic scheme, it dawned on him. Cadavers, or some particulate matter residing within them, may not be the only source of toxic particles. From the two recent cases, Semmelweis concluded that infected living beings must also produce some sort of noxious, degenerating material within their wounds not too dissimilar from cadavers. Some agent resided in diseased, decomposing tissues, whether ichorous or cadaveric in origin, which had the potential to produce the same type of pyemic ferment in the living, healthy patient.[7]

Those two unfortunate incidents also demonstrated to Semmelweis the veracity of something else: the "analogy," or causal interconnection, between erysipelas and puerperal fever, something recognized for so long in Britain, but up until now essentially ignored on the Continent. Erysipelas produced a decomposition of organic matter—in other words, ichorous material—that might then be spread to other patients by hospital personnel via their fingers, bed clothes, sponges, and so on.

While the additional deaths were tragic, Semmelweis at least learned from them. He broadened his concept of how the disease originated. Since puerperal infection could be caused by either toxic cadaveric sources or ichorous material, he replaced the term "toxic cadaveric particles" with "decomposed animal organic tissue" in his infectious scheme. With Semmelweis's single amendment to his theory and his new-found respect for infected tissues incorporated into his chloride scheme, Semmelweis experienced smoother sailing. In the following year, 1848, with his regimen fully entrenched, his mortality rate sank to 1.27 percent, and for the first time, the death rates in Division II exceeded those in Division I.[8]

Semmelweis made one other fateful declaration regarding a concept that would prove to be the major cause of his grief over the course of his career. As he further contemplated his newly formed theory, he made a generalization, a gigantic heuristic leap, concerning the manner in which puerperal fever was propagated. This step would even surpass the notions of his visionary New School mentors: Every case of puerperal fever, *without exception*, occurs consequent to the resorption of decomposing animal-organic matter into genital wounds caused by labor. This idea of exclusivity eventually evolved into Semmelweis's mantra.

In a world in which scientists considered disease causation to be multifactorial, from atmospheric and telluric forces, injured modesty, psychic stress, and so on, Semmelweis's concept of exclusivity, a single causative agent, an agent that is both necessary and sufficient to cause disease, was virtually unheard of. In effect he was saying, "One specific causative agent for one specific disease." Such a concept appeared to be too extreme even for modernists such as Rokitansky, Skoda, Hebra, Chiari, and other Semmelweis supporters to accept. In this era, thirty years before the idea of bacteria was generally appreciated and the germ theory accepted as fact, such a concept, "one agent per one disease," was just too revolutionary to be acceptable.

Endogenous Sources

Semmelweis made one further point about the origin of infections. Most cases of puerperal fever (99 percent) were exogenous in origin, with contaminants originating from an outside source. However, it is also possible for infection to be endogenously sourced, that is, from a contaminant already residing within the body. Semmelweis knew that these so-called instances of autoinfection were not preventable. Therefore, despite the best of efforts, a consistent 1 percent mortality rate was the theoretical best that any caregiver might achieve.[9]

With these new revelations now publicly announced, Semmelweis next articulated, in a more formal fashion, the three steps involved in the development of puerperal fever. First, puerperal fever was an absorptive disease. Decomposed animal-organic matter was introduced into wounded tissues via the examining finger, the surgeon's hand, soiled bed clothes, linens, soiled hands of ancillary personnel, or even, in some instances, atmospheric air.[10] Absorption of this decomposed animal-organic matter incited inflammation wherever a genital injury might have occurred, whether it be the birth canal, the cervical os (mouth), or the site of placental implantation. If some patient happened to be blessed with a strong immune system, the infection might remain localized to the uterus (metritis) or tubes (salpingitis). In each of these cases, the disease would likely resolve spontaneously. However, in the more severe form, if a laceration existed, say, in the vaginal wall, the animal-organic material had free and direct access to the blood stream.

Although Semmelweis would have known that material can travel up the fallopian tubes, spreading infection into the peritoneal cavity, no one of this era appreciated how highly absorptive was the peritoneal membrane, the membrane that he had dissected so many times. It was essentially a direct line into the bloodstream. Once absorption occurred, stage two next ensued—the disintegration of blood caused by the contaminant. Whether one called it a crasis, sepsis, or pyemia made little difference. This disintegrative phase in the bloodstream then rapidly led to the third, or exudative, stage, with its volumes of milky-white liquid invading the bodily cavities. Next came the random dissemination, via the bloodstream, of septic metastases into multiple internal organs throughout the body. As a result, abscesses appeared in such organs as the kidneys, heart, lungs, brain, and so on.[11] As degeneration continued, organ failure ensued, leading to increasing fever and confusion progressing to coma and, ultimately, death.

Semmelweis's Doctrine

Finally, as a consequence of what Semmelweis had observed at the bedside, his autopsy experience, his compilation of statistics, Kollet-schka's serendipitous death, plus the two cases of ichorous infections, Semmelweis had synthesized seemingly unrelated facts and events into one major theory or doctrine. Others, such as Oliver Wendell Holmes and James Simpson, had come close to the ultimate truth by identifying some of the essential pathogenic elements of puerperal fever. However, it was only Semmelweis who ably gathered all disparate parts of the puzzle into one unifying scheme. This recitation of the three steps involved in the production of puerperal fever became his *Lehre* (teaching), or doctrine. Although Semmelweis was not commenting about other diseases in general, when it came to puerperal fever, he was resolute: one specific agent produces one specific disease—a revolutionary concept of causation. The question was, could his colleagues be convinced of this epic achievement concerning the manner in which new mothers became infected?

Hebra's Contribution

Hebra was one of the first to learn the details of Semmelweis's discovery and his ability to dramatically decrease mortality rates. He was so impressed that he suggested to Semmelweis that, if validated by others, this discovery could be every bit as momentous as Jenner's work with smallpox. Hebra urged his former student to publish his data, to speak out on the topic as early and widely as possible—a suggestion that prompted Semmelweis to utter his well-known declaration. He not only hated polemics but he had, as well, "an innate aversion to everything that could be called writing."[12] Undeterred, Hebra considered the news so urgent that, in December 1847, he took the reins himself by addressing Vienna's Society of Physicians. In his address, "Experience of the Highest Importance Concerning the Etiology of Epidemic Puerperal Fever in Lying-In-Hospitals," Hebra covered the highlights of Semmelweis's discovery, even presenting some of his pertinent statistics.[13] Staying true to Semmelweis's own ideas, he declared that not just cadaveric particles, but "other ichorous exudates of the living" could cause the disease, as well. In December 1847, his article was published in the *Journal of the Medical Society of Vienna*, the literary arm of the Medical Society of Vienna. It included the following plea for further independent observers: "In publishing these experiences we invite the Directors of all of the lying-in institutions, some of whom Dr. Semmelweis has already informed about these most important observations, to contribute the results of their investigations either to support or to refute them."[14]

Hebra's plea, unfortunately, elicited virtually no response. Undeterred, he gave a follow-up address in January 1848 concerning further experiences at the Vienna Hospital. On this occasion, he equated Semmelweis's discovery to the work of Jenner. Hebra pointed out how Semmelweis's work had not only received confirmation from local maternity homes, but a few voices had also risen from far abroad, such as Amsterdam and Kiel, certifying the correctness of the theory. Once again, Hebra closed by challenging obstetrical directors across Europe to employ the chlorine washes, collect their own data, and issue public reports on their findings. Verification of Semmelweis's work was that important. Again, Hebra was as perplexed as he was disappointed by the lack of response from obstetricians across Europe.[15]

Spread of Doctrine

Karl Rokitansky, contrary to his usual pioneering views, had believed for years that puerperal fever was a type of "fibrinous blood crasis." As he saw it, the disease was precipitated by some force more along humoral lines that produced an excess of fibrin in the blood. However, after reviewing Semmelweis's work, he soon began revising his own views on the disease, warming to its inherent logic. Ultimately, he authenticated Semmelweis's theory, giving it his formal imprimatur by describing it in his own *Handbook of Pathologic Anatomy*.[16]

While Rokitansky may not have fully understood Semmelweis's unique view regarding causation, as pointed out later, having such an early and auspicious convert in his corner should have augured well for Semmelweis and his theory. In fact, as news spread locally, nearly all New School faculty members began falling in step behind Semmelweis. Predictably, Old School members remained unconvinced. With faculty taking sides on the issue, tensions between the two factions inevitably mounted.

Revolution

As if the increasing political turmoil swirling around Semmelweis within the confines of Vienna General Hospital were not enough to keep him fully occupied, a far larger political conflagration soon supervened. In early 1848, a revolution erupted and spread across central Europe, its origins emanating from ideals of the Enlightenment and the French Revolution. Since most of the dissidents who espoused these liberal ideals and pushed for political reform resided in Vienna, Pest, and Prague, these three cities developed into the epicenter of central European tensions. This major political conflict was a macro-expression of analogous tensions going on within the field of medicine on a more microscopic scale. Whether the dissidents were politicians representing their respective countries or university faculty and students agitating for their schools on a more local level, all of these radicals shared one lofty aspiration in common: greater autonomy. The general public desired an increase in personal freedoms, such as a more liberal constitution, cessation of serfdom, freedom of religious expression, and the like, while men of medicine wanted academic freedom in all of its ramifications. Since the ideals espoused by the dissidents coincided closely with New School philosophy, Semmelweis, along with most New School members, actively supported the revolution.[1]

In March, a cadre of three thousand Vienna University students felt an efflorescent surge of power as their crowd of rebels suddenly swelled to six thousand. The students confidently demanded academic freedom from the Austro-Hungarian ministerial authorities.

In one major confrontation, dissidents managed to close down the university on March 26, 1848. Imperial ministers soon capitulated and retreated to a safer place, Innsbruck.[2] In this "springtime of the peoples," the liberals, enjoying full control, instituted constitutional reforms, a free press, a national guard, as well as other reforms. Even the chronically repressed province of Hungary gained sufficient autonomy to begin creating its own army and conducting its own foreign policy.[3] In May, Austrian students, flushed with success, coalesced into their own action league, the Academic Legion. Members donned the revolutionary garb—grey trousers, blue jacket, and wide-brimmed hat. Although the huge commitments of Semmelweis's assistantship prohibited him from participating in the demonstrations, he proudly wore the legion's conspicuous uniform. He even lectured to medical students while wearing it, much to the dismay of the pro-establishment Klein.[4]

Although dissidents won round one by gaining dominance over the empire in the spring, concessions gained by the radical politicians, students, and faculty proved short-lived. The Austrian Empire launched a counter-revolution aided by Prague's field marshal Alfred Windischgratz and, ultimately, by a cadre of 140,000 Russian troops. Prague fell to the counter-revolution in June 1848, followed by Vienna in October. In the spring of 1849, aided by the Russians, the Austrian Empire ultimately defeated the Hungarian rebels, and Austria once again established an absolutist monarchy with the Habsburgs firmly back in control.[5] As the empire declared martial law, all of the radical policies enacted by the dissidents in the spring of 1848 were ultimately reversed.[6] With the revolution squelched, the pendulum of power swung inevitably back again towards the established order. While censorship again became the order of the day, it was not as severe as it had been prior to 1848. When it came to general politics, all edicts emanated from Schonbrunn Palace, while at the University of Vienna, the conservative Old School, with its imperial connections, enjoyed a resurgence of power, an influence gained at the expense of the New School. As a consequence, the political influence of Professor Klein and his ally, Deputy Director of the Medical Faculty Anton Rosas, rose—a change that would profoundly affect the young assistant, Semmelweis.

Skoda's Role

With revolutionary activity on the wane, academic matters again resurfaced at Vienna General Hospital. Sometime in 1848, Skoda learned the details of his former student's theory and how dramatically he had reduced puerperal fever mortality rates. Like Hebra, Skoda was similarly impressed, but Skoda envisioned something more than just a revolutionary theory. Semmelweis's great generalization, his entire inductive scheme, was a prime example of New School methodology. The way Semmelweis had employed modern scientific principles in solving a medical problem had been exemplary. Skoda sensed not only a grand opportunity to advance theoretical scientific medicine, but also to improve the image of the New School at the same time. Faculty members should be made aware of how the employment of modern research methods had made this great discovery possible. In January 1849, Skoda delivered a major address to Vienna's Committee of Professors in which he celebrated his young mentee as a prime example of someone who had learned and employed the modern scientific method to solve a major enigma. He called Semmelweis's new theory "one of the most important discoveries in the domain of Medicine."[7] Skoda led his assemblage step by step along Semmelweis's path to enlightenment, accenting his use of statistics and *per exclusionem* as his primary methods of logic. In the process, Semmelweis solved an enigma that had frustrated some of the best minds of medicine for nearly a century.

Skoda's exposition to the professors was complete except for one unfortunate point of omission. He attributed the cause of puerperal fever according to Semmelweis's first iteration of the theory—the absorption of "cadaverous particles"—failing completely to mention that the theory had been expanded to include "decomposing animal-organic matter." As explained below, perhaps Skoda did not completely comprehend the full significance of his omission. While omitting the phrase "degenerating animal-organic material" might sound minor, it made the theory appear too heuristically narrow and therefore more difficult for agnostics to accept. After all, puerperal fever could be seen in certain other infectious contexts completely unrelated to cadavers, such as erysipelas, for example. Unfortunately, Skoda's flawed version of the theory, uttered by a man of such gravitas, became immutably ingrained in the minds of too many physicians.[8]

In any narrative concerning Semmelweis, Skoda's views on causation might ordinarily be but a brief aside. Yet Skoda's position concerning his former student is worth exploring further, since on the surface it can only be seen as paradoxical. According to America's authority on Semmelweis, Dr. Codell Carter, Skoda never fully agreed with Semmelweis's idea of exclusivity, that toxic material alone, whether from the dead and or the living, was the single, sufficient, and necessary cause of puerperal fever. Whenever he gave addresses on the subject of puerperal fever, he referred not to the cause, but rather the "causes" of the disease. In October 1846, fully six months before Semmelweis unveiled his great discovery, Skoda delivered a medical school lecture formally expressing his long-held belief that disease causation was a multifactorial phenomenon. "Correct theories can only be introduced into medicine by men who give up the haughty pretension of deriving all appearances from one fundamental principle," he stated.[9] Even in the latter 1850s, when lecturing on the general subject of fevers, Skoda still referred to such causes as "chilling, overheating, over-filling the stomach, bad food, dietary errors . . . powerful emotional forces, miasmata and contagia . . . and finally mechanical disturbances."[10] There is no evidence that Skoda ever split from orthodoxy, remaining a committed multicausalist throughout his career.

Yet, recognizing how successful Semmelweis's preventive regimen had been, how could he, as a modernist, not accept the theory? The dramatic decrease in mortality rates was *prima facie* evidence that Semmelweis's theory had been built on solid ground. The success of the program spoke for itself. Skoda thus had to tread a narrow line between exclusivity and multicausalism. He never uttered any specific public condemnation of Semmelweis's contention, his "one cause for one disease" idea. And, his clearest, most definitive statement of support of Semmelweis came in 1849, two years after elucidation of the theory. In that lecture, Skoda stated that Semmelweis had "discovered the true cause of the unusually high morbidity in the first clinic and the means of reducing it to the usual level." Did Skoda not fully understand his junior's position concerning the cause(s) of puerperal fever, or did he choose, for a more overarching political reason, to remain silent on that particular aspect of causation? From a practical standpoint, Semmelweis's chloride regimen was so concrete and convincing, so effective, why should Skoda be bothered by some intangible rhetorical inconsistencies regarding how many causes there were to a disease?

Whatever his reasons may have been, Skoda treaded that narrow line, speaking in favor of the *Lehre* while continuing to believe in multicausalism. For Skoda and his war on the medieval Old School, Semmelweis's triumphant elucidation of the puerperal fever question represented too great an opportunity to squander over some theoretical disagreement. Better to just push heuristic disagreements to one side. Skoda was thus able to remain one of Semmelweis's most avid supporters during the younger man's entire stay in Vienna.

While Skoda's addresses helped Semmelweis gain greater exposure for his new theory, his efforts, on balance, proved more harmful than beneficial to the cause. Semmelweis never made any effort to correct Skoda's mistaken reference to cadaveric material being the cause of puerperal fever, resulting in incalculable damage to the theory. In addition, Skoda's celebration of Semmelweis's methods and his epic accomplishment undoubtedly exacerbated the tensions between Semmelweis and Klein.[11]

While Skoda's suggestion of a select committee to the Committee of Professors may have been a desirable move for medicine and the hospital, it added to Semmelweis's high profile pro-revolutionary, New School sentiments, thereby increasing tensions between him and Klein, a tenuous relationship in no need of further exacerbations. In fact, as biographer Sinclair claimed, Semmelweis's open support of the revolt alone had a "disastrous influence" on the young man's career.[12] Still, Semmelweis looked forward optimistically to March 20, 1849, since it marked the two-year anniversary of his assistantship. Feeling confident that his research was headed in the right direction, his hopes remained high for another two-year assignment—two years that would allow him to tie up some loose ends of his research and burnish his *Lehre* into its final form. Semmelweis had no reason to be pessimistic about his reappointment. His predecessor, Breit, and his colleague in Division II both received extensions. Another two-year appointment seemed a certainty. Yet, when he approached Klein, the professor turned him down, effectively firing him. Klein lied, offering the excuse that, as a rule, assistants only received single two-year assignments. Suddenly faced with unemployment once again and having no desire to leave the university, Semmelweis immediately applied to Klein for an alternative position, that of private docent in practical obstetrics. In that job, he would still have privileges at the lying-in hospital and he could wind up his research. Klein kept Semmelweis waiting until April, at which time he declined Semmelweis's application. Incredibly, Semmelweis applied for the same position a second time at a later date.

In October 1849, with the political waters somewhat less turbulent, Skoda delivered a second address on Semmelweis's theory, this time to the highest scientific body in Austria, Vienna's Academy of Science. After covering essentially the same points as he had in his first address, Skoda concluded by recommending that the Vienna Medical Faculty appoint an *ad hoc*, formal commission to study, in detail, all aspects of the disease, search for new or substantiating patterns of causation, and confirm further the validity and practical value of Semmelweis's new doctrine. Skoda recognized that any formal study by a committee would inevitably contrast, in bold face, the New School's modern methodology against the archaic theories and methods of the Old School. After a contentious vote, the majority of the faculty accepted Skoda's proposal and duly appointed the commission. But when Klein discovered that he had been excluded from membership on the committee, he was thoroughly insulted by the very existence of such a plan. Already feeling threatened by Semmelweis and his revolutionary doctrine, Klein rose up in opposition. Any investigative committee such as this would likely lay bare any and all dysfunction within his department. It could prove to be a huge indictment of his entire body of work. Why should such a committee be able to air Klein's dirty linen in public? Should he not have some control, some voice about what went on in his own department?[13] But Klein was not the only one placed in a tenuous position. Skoda, never an expert on interpersonal relationships, had placed his rhetorically reticent young protégé in an equally difficult position. By holding Semmelweis and his theory up as an example of modern scientific effort, Skoda had placed him at the center of this heightened debate, face to face with Klein, even as Semmelweis was awaiting Klein's decision on his docent application.

The entire affair caused even deeper schisms within the already-fractured Vienna faculty. Old School reactionaries attacked Skoda personally, charging that he was, in reality, launching an attack on Klein's personal honor under the pretense of scientific inquiry. If any investigations were to be done, they should be under the direction of Professor Klein.[14] Seeing the proposal as an open declaration of war, Klein appealed to Deputy Director Anton Rosas. Klein had one big advantage at this point. One year after the revolution, tensions between the Old and New Schools remained highly charged. With the resurgence of Austro-Hungarian imperial authority, both he and Rosas could generally count on the backing of the powerful ministerial authorities. In fact, the ministry had just conveniently promoted Rosas, a stalwart *de facto* leader of the Old School, to his new post of deputy director of the faculty.[15] Predictably, Rosas ruled in Klein's favor, and the committee never met. But that hardly diminished tensions between the two schools. Even after the decision had been rendered, heated confrontations continued between the conservatives, Klein and Rosas, and the radicals, Rokitansky and Skoda. Skoda, in particular, repeatedly left himself open to attack by faculty members on behalf of Semmelweis.[16]

Whatever Skoda's views might have been concerning mono- or multicausality, he had great faith in Semmelweis's chloride regimen, given its obvious successes. Following his addresses to Vienna's Academy of Science, Skoda published an article in the *Vienna Medical Journal*, in which he innocently created yet another firestorm. In the innocent hope of spreading the beneficent effects of the chloride regimen in correcting a well-known and long-festering problem, he made an unsolicited and unwanted recommendation to some colleagues, whom he identified in his article. It was no secret that the puerperal fever mortality rate in Prague's maternity clinic was even more dismal than it was in Vienna. With one clinic designed exclusively for physician training, and another for midwives, Prague's general set-up was much the same as Vienna's. The ever-impolitic Skoda suggested that Prague's clinic, under Wilhelm Scanzoni, its private docent, adopt chloride washings as a means of stemming their raging mortality rate. But Skoda had badly misread

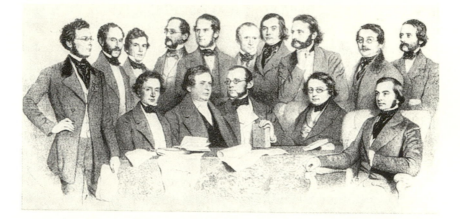

Figure 17. The University of Vienna medical faculty of 1853. Sitting, left to right: Schuh, Rosas, Rokitansky, Skoda, and Dumreicher. Standing, left to right: Hyrtl, Sigmund, Redtenbacher, Unger, Haller, Brucke, Oppolzer, Helm, Hebra, and Dlauhy.

the proud and ambitious Scanzoni who, despite his youth (he was three years junior to Semmelweis), already enjoyed some renown. He had previously made his position on puerperal fever known in an 1846 article, when he declared that a fibrinous crasis of the blood was the *condition sine qua non* for puerperal fever—all ultimately consequent to miasmatic-cosmic-telluric influences. "By no means is the wound of the uterus, represented by the placental site, the real cause of origin of the puerperal fever," he stated.[17]

Enraged by Skoda's audacious offering of unsolicited advice, Scanzoni directed his anger more at Semmelweis, creator of the message, rather than Skoda, the messenger. Scanzoni claimed that the entire theory about absorbing cadaveric particles and chloride washings was of minimal importance. As to Semmelweis's assertion that puerperal fever is just another type of pyemia—ridiculous! Furthermore, Scanzoni claimed that during one Prague epidemic, not only had he discontinued all dissections, but he had even given the chloride regimen more than a two month trial.[18] The epidemic ceased spontaneously in May, well after the chloride washes had been terminated. Clearly, chloride had been of no value. If the malady were really contagious, Scanzoni contended, "then all the lying-in-hospitals must be considered state-supported murder-dens."[19] It was, in fact, the *Genius epidemicus* that had forced the epidemic to a halt by the changes it wrought upon cosmic-telluric-miasmatic conditions. For a man even younger than Semmelweis, Scanzoni's theorizing sounded more like a seventeenth-century student of Sydenham than anything like a modern Skoda.

Tension between Vienna and Prague dissipated somewhat when Scanzoni left Prague upon the death of Professor Kiwisch, to assume the latter's prestigious chair at Wurzburg. There, with time, Scanzoni gained recognition as Germany's foremost obstetrician.[20] Scanzoni refused to reexamine his views for more than a decade, stubbornly adhering to his "crasis" theory until 1867. According to Waldheim, this early disagreement between Semmelweis and Scanzoni festered over years, finally degenerating into a personal, hateful contretemps poorly disguised as a scientific exercise.

With Scanzoni's departure for Wurzburg, his successor, Bernard Seyfert, was left to carry on the battle with Semmelweis. In full support of Scanzoni, Seyfert claimed no correlation existed, salutary or otherwise, between chloride washings and puerperal fever. In fact, virtually all obstetricians in Prague agreed that epidemics, in perfect concurrence with the epidemic view, increased in the cold winter months, before improving in warmer summer months. Seyfert then continued the party line by declaring, "Chlorine as a disinfectant seems to us an *arcanum*." Finally, it is surprising to learn that Skoda finds puerperal fever to be "the same disease as pyaemia . . . Endometritis [uterine infection] does not in any way belong to the characteristic symptoms of puerperal fever." Late in 1850, Scanzoni chimed in yet again in full support of Seyfert when Scanzoni published another paper declaring that "the conveyance of cadaveric poison as a cause of puerperal fever is an erroneous and arbitrary statement."[21]

Yet, those who had studied under Semmelweis at the time of his discovery, or had at least been associated with the hospital to witness the beneficent effects of the prophylaxis regimen, were staunch supporters. One young trainee, Friedrich Wieger of Strasbourg, had studied under Semmelweis just as chloride washings were being instituted. Weiger became so convinced of the doctrine's validity that he resolved to make it known generally in France. He began by explaining the theory to his own mentor, Professor Stoltz, only to be promptly rebuffed. The theory was utter nonsense. Undeterred, Weiger published an article, in 1849, on the cause and prophylaxis of puerperal fever in the *Union Medicale*. The *Union*'s agnostic editors placed his essay in the "doubtful anecdotes" section. Angered by such treatment, Weiger requested that Semmelweis send a communiqué to the Academy of Science. It, too, was ignored.[22] Facing up to reality, Weiger had to admit that Semmelweis's *Lehre*, at least in eastern France, would be a difficult sell.

During this same period, another foreigner who had studied in Vienna, C. H. F. Routh, delivered Semmelweis's message, in 1848, to the Royal Medical-Surgical Society of London. Upon his departure from Vienna, another student, Hector Arneth, spoke at the Academy meeting in Paris, and later, in 1850, at the Medico-Chirurgical Society of Edinburgh. Virtually all of these efforts fell, unfortunately, upon deaf ears, save for one prominent convert. England's James Simpson, despite his earlier resistance, finally became convinced that Semmelweis's doctrine was valid after hearing Arneth's convincing presentation of the facts.[23]

Still caught in the position of treading that narrow line, speaking in favor of his theory while avoiding any exacerbations with Klein, Semmelweis was met with an attractive, yet anxiety-inducing offer. Carl Haller, Vienna General Hospital's medical director, would innocently exacerbate tensions further between mentor and mentee even as Semmelweis awaited his chief's decision concerning his docent appointment.

Semmelweis Speaks

While preparing his annual hospital report in February 1849, Dr. Karl Haller, deputy director of Vienna General Hospital, could not help but be impressed by a simple fact. Division I mortality rates for 1848 were approximately one-sixth of what they had been in each of the preceding twelve years. After some investigation, he finally connected the lower mortality rates to Semmelweis's chloride regimen. Such a dramatic improvement in patient outcomes both impressed Haller and made him a near-instant convert to Semmelweis's theory. Imploring the young assistant, he declared that it would be a shame if Semmelweis did not present his epochal work to the Medical Society. "The importance of this experience for lying-in-hospitals and for hospitals generally speaking . . . is so immeasurable, that it appears worthy of the attention of all men of science."[1] Semmelweis considered it a great compliment to address a body as august as the Medical Society. Yet, he knew that his revelations would represent a huge threat to Klein. Any address would be viewed as one more major rebuke, nothing but a further condemnation of the professor and his department. When Klein finally did receive word of Haller's invitation to Semmelweis, it was, predictably, just too much for the threatened Klein to bear. On March 20, 1849, he terminated Semmelweis's assistantship.

Semmelweis was crushed by the decision. He had aimed to use the additional time for tying up some loose ends of his research and burnishing his doctrine into its final form. He hastily appealed to the dean's office, stating that his continuation as assistant was essential to the completion of his research. In addition, he asserted

that Carl Braun, his reputed successor in Division I, was not quali-
fied for the job. Having completed only two weeks on the obstetrics
ward, his was not exactly a glowing résumé. How could he manage a
large, active maternity service when he had virtually no experience?
But the stolid Klein held all the cards. His old ally, Rosas, again
came to his rescue, declaring that Semmelweis had "autocratically"
imposed his chloride washings onto the department. Klein had also
testified earlier that the washings had proven to be of "no practical value." Furthermore, with all of the friction between Klein and
his disruptive young aide, Rosas reasoned, it could be harmful to
the clinic for their association to continue.[2] With Rosas's decision,
Semmelweis was now safely marginalized, out of a job with no income and no way of continuing his research. But Klein was not quite
through with his "uncontrollable" assistant.

As previously mentioned, it was shortly after his March termination that Semmelweis applied, incredibly, for the private docent
position. Being within the same obstetrical department, the position
was, of course, controlled by Klein. How could Semmelweis have
hoped for any positive outcome when he was in an impossible position? If he did present his research to the Medical Society, Klein
would see it as an unpardonable airing of the department's imper-
fections to all Medical Society members. As Semmelweis waited
passively, hoping for appointment as docent, he was the supplicant,
relying on the mercies of the very same Klein whom he was critiquing. Klein, no doubt savoring the anguished position in which he
saw his former assistant languishing, would keep him waiting for
nearly one year.

Semmelweis's Address

With the threatening specter of Klein hanging over him on the one
hand, and hopes of overcoming the inexplicably passive attitude
of his colleagues towards his theory on the other, the ever-reticent
Semmelweis finally came to a fateful decision. He would speak out
in defense of his theory. On May 15, 1850, more than a year after
his termination, he formally addressed the Society of Physicians on
"The Origin of Puerperal Fever." As the day arrived, Semmelweis
discovered that Rokitansky, now rector of the university, would pre-

side over the meeting.[3] Records are not clear, but Klein was almost certainly in the audience. How could he miss such a major critique of his own department?[4] Could Semmelweis hew that narrow line—making his points forcefully while, at the same time, avoiding any offense to Klein?

Semmelweis began his address dispensing with the majority of existing, archaic theories of causation, such as overcrowding, weakness of spirit, embarrassment, miasmatic conditions, and the like. He paid tribute to the great accomplishments of Professor Boer, whose mortality rates for his entire tenure, 1789 to 1822, varied only a fraction above or below 1 percent. To make the next point, a comparison of mortality rates during the tenures of Boer and the unnamed Klein, Semmelweis did not have to mention either professor by name. By merely referring to mortality rates of a particular era, such as 1823 to 1826, the audience was very aware of who occupied the obstetrical chair during that particular era. Semmelweis demonstrated how, after 1822, which was the year that Klein assumed Boer's professorship, on some occasions, nearly "one patient out of every two" died of puerperal fever. Compared to Boer's average mortality of 1 percent, this was devastating news to have aired in public.[5]

Speaking with minimal notes since he had such command of the subject, Semmelweis then progressed to his main point: Puerperal fever develops when putrid animal-organic material, whether from the dead or the infected living, enters the bloodstream of the mother, resulting in a degenerative ferment within the blood. Puerperal fever is not a disease *sui generis*. It is rather just another form of pyemia, a ferment which, in turn, results in both generalized exudates and metastatic abscesses throughout the body.[6] Placing a major stress on prophylaxis, he pointed out how easily caregivers could spread the disease via the examining finger, by hands, surgical instruments, dirty linens—even through polluted air. Semmelweis delivered his points with surprising conviction. Despite his prior claims of fearing public exposition in any form, he had comported himself well.

His address was so well received that the Medical Society planned two additional meetings for 1850, one in June and a second in July. Both meetings were designed more in dialectic form, to allow for the expression of opposing viewpoints. Two adherents of the miasmatic theory would argue against Semmelweis—Eduard Lumpe and Franz Zipfl. The first, Lumpe, Division I assistant in 1840 to 1842, argued that puerperal fever clearly could not have a single cause. Its incidence varied too much with the seasons.[7] Lumpe later wrote *A Theory of Puerperal Fever*, in which he admitted to being pleased when he first heard of Semmelweis's chloride regimen, even though he had his doubts. He then asserted the counterintuitive: when he was Division I assistant, cases of puerperal fever were more numerous in the months in which he did not work on cadavers. So, how could some kind of cadaveric toxin be causally related to puerperal fever?[8] Furthermore, it was inconceivable to him that an examining finger could be the principle carrier of infection. While stopping short of labeling the chloride regimen a waste of time, he wondered how a regimen so simple—the mere application of a chemical—could solve a problem that had stumped some of medicine's greatest minds for centuries. Yet, in front of such a learned audience, Lumpe was wise enough to avoid going too far out on a limb. Playing both ends for the middle, he prudently recommended that obstetricians should, in effect, wear both belts and suspenders. Until more information comes forth they should both "wait and wash."[9]

The second speaker, Franz Zipfl, prior assistant in Division II, was a notoriously active dissector. Despite experiencing mortality rates as high as 10 to 15 percent, he openly refuted any connection between his performance of autopsies and his infection rates. Yet, he was unable to offer any tenable alternative regarding either the cause or prevention of childbed fever.[10]

There were other speakers, such as Franz H. Arneth, former student under Semmelweis, who expressed strong agreement with the cadaveric infection theory. Theodore Helm, another obstetrical assistant in Vienna, declared that no one had ever delineated so clearly the cause of this scourge as had Semmelweis. Helm placed more hope in the preventive aspects of the doctrine, since no definitive treatment was available.

As the third meeting concluded, Rokitansky declared the entire effort a perfect triumph for Semmelweis and his doctrine. But Semmelweis had committed one big error of omission, something seemingly congruent with his personality. Speakers invited to address the

Medical Society were expected to submit their notes at meeting's end for publication in the society's *Transactions*. Despite his great oral presentation, Semmelweis had not bothered to prepare any formal written notes. As a result, his first opportunity to have his groundbreaking work published in a prestigious journal amounted to nothing more than a summary of his address.[11]

Despite his trouble with the written word, Semmelweis still maintained great faith that his theory would spread easily throughout the greater medical community with just a modicum of effort. With the facts so obvious and the message so vital to humankind, how could it not? Like Shakespeare's Launcelot, he had faith that, inevitably, "the truth will out."[12] But in a medical world still dominated by archaic humoral theory, Semmelweis's doctrine was just too extreme to swallow. It threatened the very foundations of the sacrosanct cosmic-telluric-miasmatic theory and *Genius epidemicus* pounded into the heads of medical students for hundreds of years. How could some invisible, single contaminant be the one and only, immediate and necessary, cause of it all? Accepting such a theory required a total rejection of their comfortable, multifactorial views of causation. The entire theory was too radical a departure from contemporary theory. One might not be surprised to find those of Klein's generation deeply agnostic to the theory, but even many of the recently educated Semmelweis contemporaries, who had trained at less enlightened universities than Vienna's, had difficulty working it into their own theoretical schemes.[13] In addition, guilt on the part of the physician played a major role in resisting this new notion. The thought that they, as caretakers, might be spreading such a horrible disease was just too much to bear. Any accoucheur who might subscribe to such a theory would owe a major *mea culpa* to the public, something most practitioners seemed unwilling to do.

As tensions continued, Semmelweis was still awaiting Klein's decision regarding his second application. But Klein saw no reason to rush his decision. He had the ability to leave Semmelweis dangling for months. Like it or not, the professor held absolute power over his upstart assistant. Comfortable with the notion that he could count on Old School backing whatever his actions, he was in no mood to make a quick decision.

Termination

Finally, on October 10, 1850, Klein decided to act on Semmelweis's long-pending application. In what amounted to little more than a cynical trick, Klein did not fire Semmelweis. Instead, he granted him an appointment in theoretical, rather than practical, obstetrics. While the title might have sounded significant enough, in fact, it meant a low-ranking, unpaid position. He would be expected to lecture five days per week. Ignoring what this gifted man might have to offer students clinically, the position would not allow Semmelweis to have any patient care responsibilities at all. He could not even attend deliveries. While he was permitted to teach the mechanics of delivery, he was restricted to using the leather mannequin exclusively—no contact with cadavers allowed.[14]

As he contemplated his most recent loss, Semmelweis was devastated. Finally, he was fully marginalized, powerless, essentially emasculated. With his research base gone and no means of earning a livelihood, for Semmelweis, the appointment was worse than outright termination.

But Klein, with his motivations so transparent, had to endure his own sort of opprobrium, both from colleagues as well as from individuals outside the university. One such critic was Adolf Kussmaul, Semmelweis's faithful convert. He openly called Klein a "mediocre practitioner, raised to his position through influential friends," rather than on the basis of professional merit.[15] Even outside of Austria, the renowned French obstetrician, H. Varnier, exclaimed, "It is to the discredit of Professor Klein that he cut short the impetus of Semmelweis, throwing back by at least twenty years the advance of one of the greatest achievements of the century."[16]

Semmelweis had a right to be deflated, yet, looking back, in spite of his own reticence, he had garnered a great deal of exposure for his new doctrine in a short period of time. While it is undeniable that the theory's originator was a poor spokesman for his own cause, still, he had practically demonstrated many times over just how efficacious his chloride of lime regimen was in preventing puerperal fever. Even for those unwilling or unable to examine the issue objectively, that success should count for something. Considering the multiple detailed expositions of his theory, delivered over a three-

year period, by him and such renowned surrogates as Hebra and Skoda, Semmelweis seemed to be off to an auspicious beginning, despite
his losses to Klein. He had made his discovery in the mecca of European medicine with the entire nucleus of the New School behind
him. He could even claim prestigious converts like Rokitansky and,
outside of Vienna, the likes of Simpson in Scotland and Michaelis in
Keil. All of their conversions should have served as a powerful force
for spreading the word. How could the physicians of Europe, Austria
and Germany in particular, fail to embrace such a lifesaving theory? Surely it would be just a matter of time before he could muster
sufficient forces to raise the level of enlightenment in the greater
European medical community—or so one might think. That is why
Semmelweis's next step proved so surprising.

Budapest

Disappointed, disheartened, and dispirited, Semmelweis discussed his immediate plans with no one. Five days after receiving Klein's devastating news, he merely gathered his meager belongings and exited Vienna for his native Budapest. No one knows Semmelweis's motivations in leaving Vienna for certain, but clearly he had to have believed that the influence of the reactionary Old School was greater than that of the New School. Semmelweis recalled how the imperial ministry had, fifty years earlier, driven Auenbrugger, Gall, and other pioneers from Vienna to Paris for having the temerity to practice such "dangerous" arts as percussion and neuroanatomy. And, he realized that the contemporary medical culture in Vienna remained less than meritocratic. Did he not see a similar fate for himself? Many years later, Adolf Kussmaull, present through much of this controversy, supported this view when he commented on Vienna's repugnant system of favoritism in his *Youthful Memories*: "there were incompetent professors and chief physicians who owed their appointments to the patronage of distinguished petticoats and influential cowls."[1] Old friend Markusovsky, already settled in Budapest, supported this notion, as well, claiming that it was Vienna's "stifling atmosphere on the scientific revolution." The New School could not stand up to the powers of the Ministry of Culture. Hoping for a better future, Semmelweis "settled down in his native country in order to pursue his scientific studies."[2]

As Semmelweis sat back in Budapest, ruminating about his future, his wounds may have been soothed somewhat when members of the Vienna Medical Society, dominated by New School members, expressed their continuing belief in him by electing him to their membership, four months after his dismissal. Fully convinced that Klein's animus and conniving would prove futile at some time in the future, they fully accepted the young protégé as "one of theirs."[3] While he must have appreciated their show of support, since he was already in Budapest, it was too late to affect his decision.

Scheurer von Waldheim, one of Semmelweis's earliest biographers, contends that Semmelweis not only did great harm to himself and his cause with his precipitous departure for Budapest, but that his move also marked the first manifestation of his mental illness. Although he gave no evidence to back up his claim, he stated, "It is very likely that this unfortunate, seemingly unmotivated decision was the first sign of the chronic mental disease of which the unfortunate Semmelweis had clearly fallen a victim."[4] When it comes to providing credible insights into Semmelweis's life, Waldheim, because of a certain familial connection, cannot be easily dismissed. His maternal aunt, Johanna, was married to the celebrated Ferdinand Hebra. Forty years after Semmelweis's death, Mrs. Hebra used to regale the young Waldheim with intimate details of the obstetrician's life.[5] Adding further evidence to Waldheim's claim that Semmelweis was already in the earliest stages of mental decline is the disparaging moniker with which some adversaries pegged Semmelweis, sometime around 1850. Whether he displayed more overt signs of mental illness than that described above, or people merely used the term to express contempt for his controversial theory, is unclear, but he was often referred to as "Pester Narr," or the "Fool of Budapest."[6]

When the New School trio received the surprising word of Semmelweis's precipitous departure, their responses varied. Rokitansky and Hebra both shook it off good naturedly. But Skoda, the one who had lifted Semmelweis from obscurity, the one who had even made enemies within the Vienna medical community for speaking up on his behalf, was not so forgiving. Believing that the young ingrate had left just as victory was within his grasp, Skoda, in essence, crossed him off forever, save for one entirely unpredictable event late in Semmelweis's life.[7] Even his valiant old friend Chiari, who had so openly declared his support for the theory in front of the Vienna Medical Society, no longer advocated for him. Continuing the repugnant culture of favoritism in Vienna, Carl Braun, a man with minimal obstetrical training, was firmly in place as assistant in Division I. Remaining forever dedicated to his own self-advancement, and to his mentor Klein, the ingratiating Braun later became professor in Vienna and was a committed Semmelweis enemy for his entire thirty-five-year tenure.[8]

Two bright spots for Semmelweis did come along in 1850, but in both cases it was, sadly, too little, too late. The first involved the aforementioned Sir James Simpson, obstetrician to Queen Victoria and longtime contagionist. In the *Monthly Journal of Medical Science*, published just as Semmelweis was leaving for Budapest, Simpson lamented the sorry situation in which mothers were consigned to premature death by the prejudiced disbelief in the contagiousness of puerperal fever by his continental brethren. He recognized that Semmelweis's measures had decreased the mortality in Vienna "immensely and immediately."[9] After initial skepticism of Semmelweis, Simpson finally declared publicly that the man was right.

The second supportive observation, already well known to Semmelweis, should have given others a new and unique perspective on the cause of puerperal fever. Alois Bednar, another Rokitansky trainee, directed the Vienna Foundling Home, located just across the street from the maternity hospital. He, like Semmelweis earlier, became aware that newborns of infected mothers died of a blood disease virtually identical to that of their mothers, with one obvious difference. Such infants exhibited no genital component in their terminal illness. Infant mortality rates in the home usually waxed and waned between 25 and 50 percent, loosely paralleling the incidence of maternal childbed fever. In monitoring those rates, Bednar noted some interesting changes, which he published in an 1850 monograph. Interestingly, infant deaths had decreased appreciably since 1847—all as a result of Semmelweis's method. Puerperal fever, Bednar proclaimed, is not only infectious, but it may be communicated to the fetus either before or during birth.[10] Just as chloride of lime can prevent the disease in the mother, it protects the infant as well. Sadly, Bednar's paper incited neither interest nor positive reaction. His reward for this diligent piece of scholarship? For thwarting orthodoxy, university officials relieved him of his influential post.

Several months after settling in Pest, Semmelweis discovered that he was a stranger in his own home town, "a broken man," bereft of family and old friends.[11] It slowly began to sink in just how devastatingly imprudent his exodus from Vienna had been, both to him and his cause. He had escaped from the comparative light of Vienna into near-total intellectual darkness. Budapest was still suffering from the political suppression that had begun decades earlier, stagnated socially, economically, and intellectually. And the sad state of affairs would not end until 1857. After Hungary was defeated in its 1848 war for independence, it became a mere appendage of Austria, in effect a police state, with strict censorship and suppression of all things political and intellectual. Since authorities allowed no medical associations or journals, enlightened medical discourse, a simple exchange of information, became impossible. Such organizations as the Society of Natural Sciences and the Congress of Hungarian Physicians and Natural Scientists, which had fostered lively discourse in the past, were all defunct.[12] As Hungarian scientist Frigyes Koranyi described the dark suppression, "Only a few of us were informed of the epoch-making events in the life of medical science, partly from Hebra's Viennese periodical, partly from the *Prague Quarterly* (*Prager Vierteljahrschrift*), and some French papers. All scientific aspiration at home was killed in the bud."[13] Semmelweis felt exiled in Budapest, and an emotional gloom matching that of his city soon enveloped him once again. He would have loved to return to the big, busy environment of a large city, Vienna in particular, but pride and a feeling that he had burned all bridges prevented any moves in that direction.[14]

By early 1851, Semmelweis had become convinced that Budapest, with all its political and intellectual repression, remained less than a nurturing environment for his research. The Habsburg Empire still maintained an iron-fisted level of repression on Hungary, a lingering remnant of the revolution. Such a political atmosphere made most efforts at intellectual activity a near impossibility.[15] Hoping for a change from such a stiflingly sterile venue, he added his name to the list of aspirants for the vacant professorship in Prague. Unfortunately, the appointment went to Johann Streng, the only applicant who proved sufficiently fluent in the Czech language.

The Balassa Circle

Nearly one year before Semmelweis's return to Budapest, one event occurred that would have a positive effect on him. In January 1850, the Medical Society of Budapest reopened, the only medical organization allowed to hold meetings. But the police surveilled all their activities, ready to censor any information they deemed unfriendly to the state.[16] As the only medical organization in Hungary, it was destined to play a vital role in both the social and scientific lives of Hungarian physicians. The society soon became dominated by the Balassa circle, an informal group composed of elite Hungarian physicians. Janos Balassa, prior activist in the revolutionary movement, had risen to the professorship of surgery at the University of Pest shortly after his release from prison. Members of Balassa's group Janos Bokai, Janos Wagner, and Lajos Markusovsky, who had moved back to Budapest four years earlier, warmly welcomed Semmelweis into their circle.[17] At one dinner gathering, with Semmelweis at the table, conversation naturally turned to puerperal fever and the current epidemic raging at St. Rochus, a local hospital on the Pest side of the river. Some present expressed doubt concerning Semmelweis's theory. Puerperal fever thrived in St. Rochus, yet no medical students trained there, and the facility conducted no autopsies. So, how could puerperal fever be related to cadavers?[18]

Saint Rochus Hospital

Intrigued, Semmelweis visited St. Rochus the next morning. True, the hospital did not train medical students, but it did not take long to identify the origin of the problem. The fault lay with the surgeon, who not only served as hospital obstetrician, but also performed forensic autopsies for the hospital. His daily routine first included rounding on the surgical ward, where infections flourished. He visited the thirty-seven-bed obstetrical floor last. He devoted his time in between these two activities to conducting autopsies. Semmelweis, sensing that he could solve this epidemiologic problem, visited the hospital supervisor, where he offered his obstetrical services without pay "for the benefit of science and the hospital."[19] After receiving his formal appointment in March 1851, he served the hospital

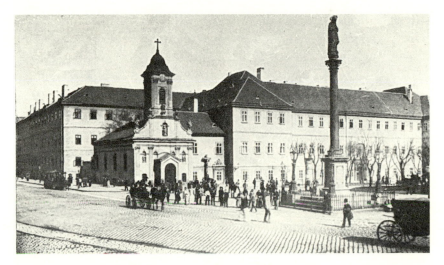

Figure 18. Budapest's Saint Rochus Hospital. Semmelweis provided all obstetrical care here for six years, free of all remuneration.

in that position, *pro bono*, for six years, a period that helped improve his dispirited state. These few years could be characterized as his happy, or at least less-unhappy, interlude. He found the hospital backward in both attitude and practices, with a poor level of general hygiene, as well as dirty bed linens and clothes, all residual influences of one Professor Birly from the nearby university. Sensing an opportunity to be of service and to perhaps propagate his theory, Semmelweis dug into his work there, implementing changes including his chloride regimen. His spirits rose as the mortality rates from puerperal fever dropped.[20] While mortality rates in Vienna and Prague were running between 10 and 15 percent, Semmelweis experienced, among 933 deliveries, only eight deaths (0.8 percent) attributable to childbed fever.[21] Not only were Semmelweis's spirits lifted, but he impressed enough people with his results that he gained some celebrated status locally.

Soon another problem raised its head in the form of finances. With the death of his mother and father, all parental largesse had disappeared. Although money never meant much to the man, he was running seriously low on funds. He, therefore, began a private practice of obstetrics and gynecology in Budapest. With his surgical expertise, his knowledge, and his natural patient rapport, he flourished medically throughout the 1850s. To his patients and to the poor, he was unerringly kind and considerate.

But those who worked around him and witnessed the manner in which he instituted his prophylactic regimen were less inclined to describe him in such benevolent terms. In fact, his old image as the felicitous one, always eager to please, had undergone a definite, yet inarticulable, evolution. Were these changes the simple summation of all his mental stresses, his trials and tribulations of the last half-decade? He lost his mother in 1844, his father in 1846, and, as a result of the failed 1848 revolution, his patriotic brothers, as well. Having been active in the revolution, they had all fled Hungary just to avoid execution. Only one sister and a brother, the Catholic priest Father Karoly, still remained in Budapest. Over six short years, 1844–1850, not only had Semmelweis witnessed the dissolution of his family, but he had also lived through the stresses of his research and the revolutionary war. On top of his depressing and demanding job as assistant, circumstances forced him to endure the hostility of his mentor, Klein, a man whose views on medical progress were antithetical to his own.

Biographers, including the aforementioned Waldheim, note that between 1849 and 1850, Semmelweis's personality had begun its subtle metamorphosis. For someone meeting him for the first time, his personality would have to be described as falling within the norm, yet to one who knew him in the early 1840s, the contrasts in personality were definite. Both his youthful, felicitous personality and his easygoing repartee had been replaced by a more serious demeanor. He had little time for frivolous, idle chatter and seemed to have lost his sense of humor. Was it a simple process of youthful maturation into that of a more serious professional who felt like he carried the world on his shoulders, or did it represent the earliest, vague stages of mental decline?

Professorship

In November 1855, Professor Ede Birly, first and only professor of Obstetrics at the University of Pest, died unexpectedly. As a search for his successor began, the influential *Vienna Weekly Medical Journal* openly advocated for Semmelweis, claiming his appointment could represent a "new epoch" in Hungarian medicine.[22] Despite this native son's prominent position in the city of Budapest, he found himself on a list with six other nominees for the chair. Adding to that humiliation, on a secret faculty ballot it was not he, but Carl Braun, who received the most votes. However, Semmelweis finally did receive the appointment, not because of his groundbreaking research, but because he spoke fluent Hungarian. In July 1856, the king officially appointed Semmelweis to his post as professor of theoretical and practical obstetrics at the University of Pest.[23]

Given his successful practice and full professorship at a mere thirty-seven years of age, one might think that Semmelweis had reached a happy pinnacle in his life, but such was not the case. In fact, his University of Pest professorship would mark the end of his happy interlude. A plenitude of insults and vexations revolving around professional autonomy, bureaucratic parsimony, archaic versus modern attitudes, were yet to come. Little improvement had occurred in Hungary's relationship with the suppressive Habsburg Dynasty and its Minister of Public Education. Overall, twelve years would transpire (1848–1860) before the monarchy allowed the university to hold general meetings, elect its own deans, or exert any sort of curricular autonomy.[24]

One of the most powerful determinants looming behind departmental policy was a severe lack of funds. The obstetrics service, located on the second floor, had only twenty-six beds, plus three in the delivery room. Unlike Vienna, where women were admitted during their final two months of gestation, in Pest they were admitted only upon inception of labor. Considering the unpleasantness of the ward, located over the malodorous hospital morgue, one could argue the briefer the confinement, the better the policy. The aroma of the privy was ever-present. Three smoke-belching chimneys arose from a chemical plant, and a nearby cemetery contributed other noxious effluents to the air. If the wind blew one way patients smelled the fetid aroma of illness; in the other it was the mixed fetor of chemicals plus putrefaction. Ward nurses had their choice: leave the windows open in the heat of summer, breathing in the blended stench of their three noxious neighbors, or close them and contend with unbearable heat.[25]

Despite Semmelweis's constant pleadings to move the ward to a more favorable location, it took a devastating hospital epidemic of erysipelas in 1859 before authorities finally acted. They moved to a facility possessing only slightly better accommodations. In these new quarters, anyone wishing to gain access to the maternity beds found it necessary to walk through the labor room. Guests, or staff carrying water, wood, both clean and dirty bedpans, and the like often found themselves intruding, unavoidably, on deliveries as they sought passage into the lying-in wards.[26]

Semmelweis's daily tasks at the university were formidable. In addition to patient care and heavy administrative duties, he was charged with teaching two hundred students annually, fifty being medical students. The remaining one hundred fifty were student midwives, virtually all from the uneducated, lower social strata. With no lecture hall, Semmelweis was reduced to addressing groups in the hallways, while students overflowed into the side corridors.

But worse than the cramped quarters facing Semmelweis was the hostile nursing staff, innocently preconditioned by Professor Birly. Despite being in Budapest and associating with the professor for five years, Semmelweis had never managed to make a convert of Birly. As a Boer trainee, Birly had long believed that puerperal fever was caused by an enlarged uterus that obstructed lower intestinal flow. His treatment consisted of purgatives and enemas. Not surprisingly, infections and high death rates had been a constant during his long tenure. As Semmelweis introduced his chloride regimen to a hospital staff conditioned to treating infected patients with Birly's regimen, he was greeted with passive aggression. Ironically, they looked upon this Hungarian patriot as a German interloper, one of the oppressors, bringing in some strange and unwanted new treatment scheme. Implementing all the little rituals connected with the chloride washings was just too much trouble. Forced to constantly monitor their less-than-enthusiastic efforts at antisepsis, each day proved a challenge for Semmelweis. The incessant resistance of hospital workers, their passive aggression, seemed to bring out Semmelweis's darker qualities. In the course of his work, when dealing with peers and subordinates whom he sensed were either antagonistic to his theory or slothful in their jobs, he had learned to not suffer such fools gladly. He had, as well, become completely indifferent to what such individuals thought of him.[27] At some point in the preceding five years, his image, if not his actual persona, had evolved into the overly-exacting, impatient, and demanding overseer. Maintaining acceptable mortality rates demanded such vigilance. Hospital staff, ignorant of the science behind Semmelweis's theory, were irked by his insistence that they adhere strictly to proper prophylactic protocol, with all its tedium. With his rigid demands, he had, to them, become the "eccentric faddist," a term whispered as he turned his back exiting the ward, and yet another moniker to add to his prior "Pester Narr."[28]

Despite such staff resistance, Semmelweis was rewarded for his assiduousness. During his first year, 1855 to 1856, he experienced only two deaths (0.39 percent) out of 514 births. Buoyed by the great results, he enthusiastically published his work, plus an updated elaboration of his theory, in the prestigious *Vienna Weekly Medical Journal*, fully expecting a great boost in the acceptance of his doctrine. But when he read the editor's remarks, "We thought that this theory of chlorine disinfection had died out long ago: . . . it would be well that our readers should not allow themselves to be misled by this theory at the present time," he was crestfallen.[29] Had his theory really died out? Perhaps he was no longer relevant.

Adding to this setback, 1856–1857 proved a bad year for Semmelweis. He lost sixteen patients to puerperal fever, a situation that sent him in all directions in search of the cause. Soon he discovered something interesting: not one of the newborns of the fatal sixteen had died. Semmelweis reasoned that it was therefore more likely the infections had occurred, not during labor, but sometime after birth, at a time too late for the newborn to become entangled in the infection. As he monitored staff activity in the labor rooms, he noticed, to his horror, that nurses were placing postpartum women directly onto malodorous, bloody, lochia-stained sheets. After a brief investigation, Semmelweis discovered that the hospital had been accepting laundry from the lowest on its list of competitive bidders, completely indifferent to quality of service. Despite his admonitions about the dangers of contamination, this antagonistic nursing staff had been deliberately flouting his rules of antisepsis. With so few allies, he would have to monitor the daily operations within the department himself if further infections were to be prevented.

Completely frustrated, Semmelweis addressed multiple letters of complaint to the hospital administrator, von Tandler. Tandler's unenthusiastic reply indicated only that "we shall investigate," in other words, sometime in the nebulous future.[30] In a fit of anger after reading the letter, Semmelweis rushed onto the ward, gathered up a pile of "fresh" linens, soiled despite having been freshly delivered from the laundry, and stormed into Tandler's office, dumping them straightaway on his desk. Faced with the filthy and aromatic "clean" sheets, Tandler not only got the message immediately, but, to his credit, he also took corrective action. While Semmelweis may have won this battle, his behavior made enemies of both Tandler and the head nurse. With the constant need to monitor and correct such churlish resistance, Semmelweis's heated, confrontational method of problem solving eventually became his *modus operandi*. With so little respect for his adversaries, the doubters around him, he became increasingly verbally abusive. His actions, compared to even five years before, were more impetuous, tactless, and alienating.

The year 1857 to 1858 proved as frustrating for Semmelweis as the previous one, when his mortality rate hit 4 percent. Investigating further, he found that several dissident nurses, in open violation of his rules, had persisted in placing women in labor on stinking sheets, soaked in the bodily fluids of predecessors. While Semmelweis managed to have all the guilty nurses fired immediately, the damage was done. Tandler sent him a letter of reprimand blaming him for the slovenly practices within his department. Hoping to avoid another confrontation with the bureaucrat, Semmelweis admitted to the substandard practices. Not blind to the irony, he did point out to Tandler that it was he who, in 1847, had discovered the cause of puerperal fever. He was the one who had actually put these very standards in place. With some soothing of Tandler's ruffled feathers, and some renewed vigilance concerning antisepsis, mortality rates once again decreased to more acceptable levels, but Semmelweis learned that he could never relax his watchfulness.[31]

Then, in 1856, word from Vienna reached Budapest announcing the death of Professor Klein, after thirty-five years at his post. Semmelweis had always harbored a hope, however distant, that he might someday be summoned to succeed his old mentor in this highest obstetrical position in all of Europe. Such an appointment would set up his triumphant return to the university. Again, he was bitterly disappointed. In a university still hostile to this "chlorine nonsense," his name did not even appear on the search committee's list. Adding to his disappointment, the position ultimately went to none other than his old nemesis, Carl Braun. Semmelweis did, however, derive some solace later in 1856, when he was offered the chair in Zurich. By that time, however, he had resolved to remain in Budapest, his cultural home.[32]

Marriage

In the midst of his continuing travails, Semmelweis did experience one bright spot in his personal life. In 1856, he met Maria Weidenhofer, twenty-year-old daughter of a prosperous Hungarian merchant. After a brief courtship, the two married in June 1857 with Father Karoly, Semmelweis's brother, conducting the ceremony. Ignaz, thirty-nine, was by now a middle-aged, corpulent professor with florid face and full coronal balding. Maria must have softened Ignaz's image to some degree in that they were socially active, attending balls and soirees, mainly under the auspices of the Medical Society.

Within two years the couple welcomed Ignaz, their first child, into the world, but soon their happiness changed to bitter disappointment. The infant died of hydrocephalus just two days after his birth. Then, in 1860, they anxiously celebrated the birth of Maria. She too, however, died tragically at four months of age. Uncertain of the exact cause, doctors attributed her death to "failure to thrive and peritonitis."[33]

Twice burned, the couple was understandably hesitant to take further chances on a third child—maybe there was something dreadfully wrong with them. However, three more healthy children did come along, with Antonia, their last, born in 1864. All three survived into adulthood. Despite the misfortunes experienced with their early family, Ignaz and Maria enjoyed a happy marriage. For Semmelweis, family life provided his singular respite from the vexations of his profession.[34]

Semmelweis became a regular reader at the library of the freshly reborn Medical Society, beginning with his earliest days in Budapest. He even managed the library formally from 1861 to 1864, during which time he organized and catalogued its entire content.

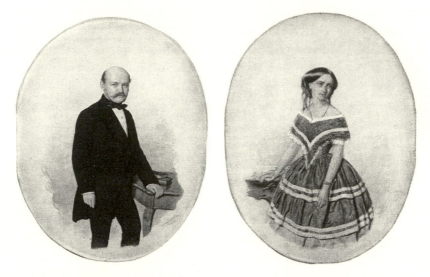

Figure 19. Paintings occasioned by the marriage of Ignaz Semmelweis, age thirty-nine, and Maria Weidenhofer, age twenty, in 1857. By Ágost Canzi (1808–1866).

Over these years he made a point of digesting all available obstetrical literature, remaining particularly vigilant for any articles on puerperal fever or any references to his doctrine in Europe. In fact, several volumes still remain in the library in which Semmelweis, unable to resist corrective editorial comments, diligently inserted his own marginalia in hopes of providing subsequent readers with a more balanced exposition.[35] While this activity clearly kept him enlightened in his field, it also served, with a few exceptions, as a chronic source of irritation and disappointment. As he scoured the journals, reading the opinions of such ill-informed "experts" in the field, his rage slowly mounted. Over the course of these eight years, he encountered a virtual fount of ignorant comments emanating from some of the putative obstetrical luminaries of Europe.

Early in his readings, Semmelweis did find some areas of brightness. The first came from former student Franz H. Arneth as he toured England, Ireland, and France. Arneth was appalled by the mortality rates in Paris, a city in which student midwives dissected alongside the medical students. In January 1851, he addressed the Academy of Medicine in Paris, outlining Semmelweis's theory and stating that "with the prophylactic method recommended by

Semmelweis it had been possible to stop the spread of the puerperal epidemic in the obstetrical hospitals of Vienna."[36] Although dubious of Arneth's address, academy members were receptive enough to appoint a committee, headed by Matheo Orfila, to study the issue. After due deliberation of Arneth's claims, the committee published its decision in the French *Lancet*, ruling against the theory of cadaveric infection. Members could not believe that a solution of chlorine, a simple chemical, could actually destroy cadaveric particles.[37] Sadly, the Maternité did not improve with time. Even as late as 1860–1864, out of a total of 9,886 deliveries at the Maternité, 1,226 deaths occurred, an average mortality rate of 12.4 percent.[38]

In June 1851, Arneth addressed the Medico-Chirurgical Society of Edinburgh, fully elaborating on Semmelweis's experience with preventing puerperal fever. With his full understanding of Semmelweis's work, Arneth gave one of the most accurate and definitive statements on puerperal infection: "Any fluid matter in a state of putrefaction—communicated by linen, by a catheter, by a sponge, by small particles of the placenta, even by the ambient atmosphere impregnated by the foul substances—may produce puerperal fever."[39] Of even greater importance, the spread of puerperal fever could be prevented by using the chloride regimen advocated by Semmelweis. Although not uttered by Semmelweis himself, Arneth's address served as one of the first important, readily understandable articulations of the theory. But for the Scotch, Arneth's statement apparently lacked sufficient clarity, as he changed no minds.

Wurzburg's Franz Kiwisch von Rotterau, known simply as Kiwisch, another of Germany's leaders in obstetrics, was one of the first to arouse Semmelweis's indignation. In his 1851 edition of a book on diseases of the female reproductive system, he rejected the notion of toxic decomposed organic matter. That idea was nothing new. Puerperal fever was miasmatic in origin—its epidemic nature was beyond question. Its first phase was a "diseased condition within the blood." All subsequent local inflammations in the body eventuated from that blood crasis. Kiwisch had obviously not altered his views as he became more experienced, since he openly admitted to performing autopsies immediately before attending to deliveries. He claimed never to have seen bad consequences from this practice.

Kiwisch did admit to one truth. He had endured a frightful epidemic in 1846 in which his mortality rate reached 26 percent, but since it persisted until the warmer time of the year, it was easy to see that atmospheric conditions were the cause. In fact, all of his repetitive outbreaks had coincided with such changes in the weather. Although a firm believer in multiple causes of puerperal fever, Kiwisch was not above playing both ends for the middle, by recommending that physicians avoid contaminating gravid women with decomposed animal material.[40] He recommended that practitioners follow both the English measures of fumigation, as well as the chloride washings as recommended by Semmelweis. Sitting in his library, Semmelweis must have fumed as he read such duplicitous comments. Kiwisch saved face by arguing against the antiseptic method on theoretical grounds, yet he silently adopted Semmelweis's methods in his own practice.[41] Kiwisch would hardly be the last to embrace this strategy.

In 1853, Scanzoni reappeared, publishing an edition of his *Manual of Midwifery* (*Lehrbuch der Geburtshilfe*), which included a section on childbed fever. In it, he took credit for being the first to cast doubt upon Semmelweis's theory that pus and ichor are produced in the blood exclusively by cadaveric particles. While he allowed that some cases of infection might possibly occur in this manner, *Genius epidemicus* was by far the most important factor. That fact was beyond dispute. "We are still of the opinion that it is [sic] chiefly miasmatic influences . . . which are at the root of the disease, most particularly, atmospheric influences. In other words, the epidemic nature of the evil cannot be denied."[42]

Some of Semmelweis's perceived literary affronts occurred by way of omission. In 1854, Eduard Lumpe included an extensive section on puerperal fever in his *Compendium of Practical Midwifery* without even mentioning the Semmelweis Doctrine. Had he really slipped so drastically that he was no longer relevant? Worse, Lumpe wrote a detailed discussion on the causes of puerperal fever that was riddled with error throughout and included a statement on the "ineffectiveness" of chloride washings.[43]

And then there was Semmelweis's successor, Carl Braun. Upon assuming his assistantship in March 1849, he referred to Semmelweis's theory as "all humbug" when lecturing to students. But, as he saw his own clinic mortality rates rise, Braun's jealousy and resentment of Semmelweis grew stronger. Just as with Scanzoni, the fight became personal for Braun, based more upon hatred and ignorance than scientific differences. In an 1854 publication, *On the Puerperal Process*, Braun further maligned Semmelweis's theory with untruths, stating, "In Germany, France and England this hypothesis of cadaveric infection has been up to the most recent time almost unanimously rejected."[44]

Enlisting others to his side, Braun asserted that five years had passed since the theory was first published and, still, those authorities possessing the most knowledge of maternity hospitals, such as Scanzoni, Lumpe, Kiwisch, and the entire Academy of Medicine in Paris, continued to deny that the doctrine had any merit.[45]

Nor was Braun above taking advantage of erroneous statistics if they favored his argument. He knew of certain clinics in which antisepsis had been practiced with enough inexactitude to cast doubt on their results. Still, as long as those authors attributed the causes to overcrowding, poor ventilation, and miasmatic air, Braun did not hesitate to cite their results, since they bolstered his own argument.[46] Then, in 1855, Braun wrote a section on puerperal fever in a collaborated handbook of obstetrics. Detailing his own contemporary ideas, he devoted forty-five pages to identifying thirty different causes of puerperal fever. Semmelweis's "cadaveric infection" barely made the list at number twenty-eight. Braun stubbornly held on to his multicausalist opinion until at least 1881.[47]

Semmelweis took great heart when reading the opinions of the iconic German chemist, Justus von Leibig, who was only peripherally involved in the puerperal fever debate. In his *Chemical Letters* of 1851, he lamented how poorly received this "great, practical, important discovery" had been. Leibig asserted that cadavers can decompose to such a degree that their poisons can infect the living. He stated, "Certainly nervous causes of puerperal fever have been seen but that which has been discovered by Dr. Semmelweis, with all the acumen of an unbiased investigator . . . cannot be doubted by an unprejudiced man."[48] But such men were either not reading, were paying insufficient attention, or clearly did not understand this unbiased investigator.

In 1857, Anselm Martin directed Munich's modern, clean, and well-ventilated Royal Maternity Hospital, a facility studiously built to control all factors considered important in the genesis of puerperal fever, such as overcrowding, filth, proximity to sources of miasmatic air, and the like. Despite such precautions, Martin's facility became the site of an epidemic that raged from December 1856 until June 1857. In a monthly obstetrics journal, Martin confidently rejected Semmelweis's doctrine outright, without citing any evidence, maintaining that the epidemic in his clinic was contagious, and not cadaveric in origin. Chloride washings were a waste of time.[49]

A bittersweet sign of support for Semmelweis occurred in early 1858 when he received a comforting letter from former student, Joseph Steiner. When Steiner moved back to Gratz to complete his medical studies, he found "infection all over their maternity hospital." Students used the dissecting rooms as their social gathering place, while making no efforts at washing. They often proceeded from morgue directly to labor rooms, "waving their bloody hands in the air." "The patients might as well be delivered in the dissecting-room," he declared. Even the medical officer of Gratz lamented that their maternity hospitals were "really nothing but murder institutions!"[50] While Steiner's support gave Semmelweis some comfort, the utter ignorance of the Gratz students and obstetrical staff was dispiriting.

France, plagued for years with high rates of puerperal infection, was no better. Impassioned but unenlightened debates, particularly in Paris, had been an ongoing fête for more than a decade. Then, in February 1858, after a distressing death of a young woman from septic abortion, members of the French Academy of Medicine convened to address the entire question of puerperal fever. Their meetings extended over seven months. Since the academy promised to publish their proceedings in multiple languages, many throughout Europe eagerly awaited their conclusions. One early speaker, Professor Jean A. H. Depaul, posed four questions to be addressed by the academy: Was there a general malady that might be designated puerperal fever? Of what did it consist? What treatment measures were of value? What means could be employed to prevent it? Answering his own queries, Depaul declared the disease contagious. Although strongly analogous to septicemia, the malady was neither a pyemia nor a septicemia. Since no treatment existed for the disease, prevention remained the only solution. Depaul's only suggestion—build smaller hospitals.[51]

Another speaker, Paul Dubois, France's most prominent accoucheur, criticized Semmelweis directly, stating that, "This opinion is no longer supported in Germany." If the disease was contagious, it was not constant, active, or persistent, otherwise all hospital personnel should be in quarantine. In a later address, Dubois claimed that the condition of puerperal fever existed before labor in a "certain number of cases," an epidemic brought to the Maternité by women already exhibiting "the most serious symptoms of puerperal fever."[52]

Dubois's colleague, Antoine Danyau, assistant surgeon at the Maternité was convinced that the disease was of miasmatic origin. Claims that the disease was transmitted "by the medical attendant, as mentioned by Semmelweis of Vienna, are not convincing, and appear to have found few supporters in Germany." One described the disease as a "local inflammation," while others admitted to some indefinable "primitive alteration of the blood," "miasmatic," "transmission by the medical attendant," and so forth. Dubois again intervened at a later meeting postulating that the disease was "produced under epidemic influence. . . . I admit the primitive alteration of the blood by a cause yet unknown . . . is the only one [theory] which I am able to accept."[53]

The more France's leading accoucheurs publically pontificated, the more clear it became that there were nearly as many theories of causation as there were speakers. No single argument proved all that compelling. Even though the answer had been evident for ten years, most attendees remained sadly confused. Since members could reach no meaningful consensus on the nature of the disease, their long awaited publication proved anticlimactic. One frustrated medical writer, Dr. Auber, commented sarcastically about the "chaotic mixture" of opinions: "Among the thirteen academicians whom we have heard, we can count essentialists, demi-essentialists, essentialists against their will, essentialists without their knowledge, absolute localizers, half and quarter localizers, localizers with a leaning towards essentialization, and essentialists with a love of localization, specifists, tyhphists, traumatists, and neo-traumatists."[54] In the decade since Semmelweis had enunciated his *Lehre*, academy members still expressed their ignorance with the greatest of confidence. Clearly, in ten years, nothing had changed at all.

Then, in April 1859, an article by Otto Franque, assistant to Scanzoni, proved particularly galling to Semmelweis. Franque described a recent epidemic in Wurzburg in which thirty-three out of ninety-nine women were struck with puerperal fever. Nine died. Now, twelve years after Semmelweis's historic pronouncement, Franque, under Scanzoni's tutelage, still voiced the same tired explanations. Atmospheric influences, "caused by the *Genius epidemicus*," were to blame for the epidemic.[55] Semmelweis blamed Scanzoni, supposed sage of German obstetrics, for his assistant's ignorance. In a dozen years, Scanzoni had not modified his antiquated views in the least.

Another event in 1859 piqued Semmelweis greatly because of its blatant obtuseness. A Dr. Silberschmidt, another Scanzoni assistant, won the Faculty of Medicine prize in Wurzburg by writing an historical critique concerning the pathology of childbed fever as viewed by the ancients up to contemporary scientists. Silberschmidt openly refuted Semmelweis's contention that cadaveric poisoning was the prime cause of puerperal fever. With views mirroring Scanzoni's, he called chloride washings unsuccessful and essentially useless. Semmelweis sensed that the entire work was little more than a regurgitation of Scanzoni's views.

Semmelweis was painfully aware of other less prominent obstetricians, too numerous to name, who expressed similarly ill-informed opinions. When it came to understanding the cause of puerperal fever, it was all too clear; not a single new ray of sunlight had illuminated the medical landscape in more than a decade. Women and their newborns were still dying unnecessarily, at unacceptably high rates. His pique only mounted.[56]

One important event in 1857 proved important to Semmelweis in that, along with his increasing anger, it helped rid him of his aversion to all forms of exposition. Nine years after the revolution, the ministry, declaring a general amnesty, released political prisoners and relaxed many bureaucratic rules. As a consequence, a reborn *Medical Weekly* (*Orvosi Hetilap*) printed its first edition that same year under its new editor and Semmelweis friend, Lajos Markusovsky. In that cordial environment, Semmelweis's aversion "to all that is called writing" slowly dissolved. His literary catharsis produced five articles up to 1865, plus another in the *Vienna Medical Journal*, on subjects as varied as uterine fibroids, menstrual problems, and surgical management of ovarian cysts.[57]

By the autumn of that year, Semmelweis finally realized that he had heard enough from his obstetrical colleagues. No longer could he let such ignorance, omissions, inaccuracies, misinformation, and deviousness go unchallenged. Casting a sorrowful eye backwards, he realized what a terrible error he had committed by remaining silent all of these years. He owed it to the public, to the young mothers and their newborns dying needlessly at the hands of complacent, incompetent practitioners masquerading as obstetrical experts. He must seek publicity, to set the record straight. But his path would prove long, solitary, arduous, and debilitating.

Aetiology

Semmelweis's formal literary offensive began on January 2, 1858, when he delivered an epic address to the Medical Society of Budapest. Many distinguished Hungarian scientists attended his presentation, which was, in essence, a precursor to his upcoming grand opus, *The Aetiology, the Concept and the Prophylaxis of Childbed Fever*. He delivered, in all, three speeches over a six-month period. In these addresses, Semmelweis covered the same topics in a more updated version that he had previously covered in Vienna. On this occasion, he was wise enough to have prepared adequate notes, which were published later in the *Medical Weekly*. This proved to be his most rational and concise exposition of the doctrine to date. Just as with his earlier address in Vienna, reception ran the gamut from enthusiastic to indifferent to hostile. Unfortunately, with the journal being printed only in Hungarian, it received little attention outside of his native country. But Marko, for one, remained enthusiastic: "Semmelweis expounded his teaching with such conviction before our society that only a man is capable of possessing who not only can fight for its truth but vouches for it with his life. His dedication to his work was evident at the meeting of the Medical Society and it deeply moved all those present."[1]

However, Hungarian physician, writer, and Semmelweis observer Theodore Duka was less impressed than was Marko. Duka later commented on a disturbing trait he perceived in the speaker. Semmelweis could not tolerate any criticism during presentation of his work. In fact, any adverse comments concerning the theory were met with hostility. Such a reception seemed to become the new

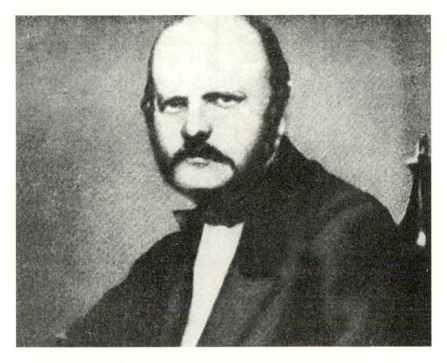

Figure 20. A sad and angry-appearing Semmelweis in 1858, age forty, as he began writing *Aetiology.*

norm for Semmelweis. Constantly preoccupied with the job at hand, he had little time for any sort of collegial exchanges or lighthearted banter with work associates. Faculty members often found their colleague to be hypercritical and intolerably punctilious, even regarding arcane academic matters. It made them hesitant to engage him in any sort of dialogue. In fact, this former smooth talking ladies' man was more often in a fighting mood. Even from a distance, one could discern a different mien. His brooding eyes revealed a painful sadness combined with a tinge of anger, as seen in Figure 20.

Looking back to 1855, Semmelweis was said to be pleasing both in character and appearance. By 1858, however, as he embarked on his writing offensive, he had become not only chronically irritable, but overtly eccentric, as well. Once impeccably attired, the man had begun dressing in an odd manner with curious choices of color and style. According to Loudon, by the time Semmelweis began writing his treatise, "it seems likely that he was in the early stages of a mental illness, the nature of which has been frequently debated and is still uncertain."[2] One other facet of his personality proved troubling. His mood, which had heretofore modulated appropriately depending upon what he encountered in his environment, became autonomous, alternating dysrhythmically from high to low, depression alternating with mania, the swings occurring without identifiable precipitating cause. According to Loudon, he suffered bouts of depression and absentmindedness, "showing signs of disorientation, interspersed with periods of manic energy and great excitement."[3]

As Semmelweis prepared for publication of his grand response to his critics, he read ever more widely, familiarizing himself in even greater depth with the literature. He also began compiling and organizing the immense amount of statistics, old and new, that he had generated through prior and ongoing research. Having monitored the journals assiduously he had an acute sense of which institutions were still suffering from the highest infection rates. Still, hoping to gain a better sense of how other obstetricians viewed the problem of puerperal fever and about how broadly accepted, or not, his *Lehre* might be in Europe, he began correspondence with some of the more prominent European professors. One correspondent, Professor Dietl of Cracow, who traveled widely, made an interesting observation. Dietl noted that many, if not most, of the institutions with which he was familiar not only avoided contact with cadavers, but had incorporated the chloride regimen into their practices, as well. They adopted these measures silently, without any sort of public pronouncement. He advised Semmelweis, "For the purposes of investigating the truth on this point a journey round the world would be well worth your while."[4] Dietl was implying something about Semmelweis's detractors, pointing out their determination, whatever their reasons, to deny Semmelweis his due.

Early biographer, Waldheim, had a definite opinion about the obstetricians' general reticence to affirm Semmelweis and adopt his methods: "They envied this man his celebrity. The vanity of the learned considered it ridiculous that this simple person, who spoke a strange dialect in his debates and scientific addresses, who had never published a single scientific contribution to obstetrics, could have made such a discovery. His accomplishment is best just simply ignored."[5] After all, how could he be right when he insisted that puerperal fever had but one exclusive cause?

In Semmelweis's introduction to *Aetiology*, he first explained the purpose for his effort. He aimed to set forth the historical observations that forced him, as a younger man, to doubt all contemporary theories of puerperal fever. In the late 1840s, his theory was proclaimed to the greater medical community not only by him but by other members of the New School. He had believed naively that, with a subject as important as puerperal fever and the cause so evident, the truth behind his theory would ultimately prevail on its own:

> But during the thirteen years, which have elapsed, my expectations have not been fulfilled to the degree which is necessary for the benefit of humanity.
>
> Misfortune ordained that in the school years 1856–7 and 1857–8 at my own obstetrical clinic in Pest the puerperae should perish in such numbers, that my opponents were able to use this mortality against me; I can show however that these two unlucky years were just many sad, unintentional, inadvertent proofs for me.
>
> To this disinclination for controversy is added an innate aversion to everything in the nature of writing.
>
> Fate has chosen me as an advocate of the truths which are laid down in this work. It is my imperative duty to answer for them. I have abandoned the hope that the importance and the truths of the facts would make all conflict unnecessary. My inclinations are of no moment alongside the life of those who take no part in the dispute over the justice of my claims or of those of my adversaries. I am constrained to come before the public once more, since my silence has been futile, and despite the many bitter hours which I have suffered, yet I find solace in the consciousness of having proposed only conclusions based upon my own convictions.[6]

Painful as it was for him to admit, up to 1858, Semmelweis's work had resulted in minimal salutary effects. Major figures of European obstetrics still referred to his doctrine as "one-sided, narrow and erroneous." His struggle was clear: to spread his doctrine to all teachers of midwifery, "Until all who practice medicine down to the last village doctor and the last village midwife, may act according to its principles . . . to banish the error from the lying-in-hospitals, to preserve the wife to the husband, the mother to the child. . . . Indignation at the greatness of this scandal has thrust the pen into my unwilling hand."[7]

One major impediment remained for Semmelweis. Before he could formally critique other obstetricians generally, he issued his second public *mea culpa*: "It would be contrary to my conscience not to confess here that only God knows the number of women whom I have consigned prematurely to the grave . . . however painful and depressing the recognition may be, there is no advantage in concealment; if the misfortune is not to be permanent, the truth must be brought home to all concerned."[8]

What Semmelweis produced in writing *Aetiology* was, in essence, an elaboration of his *Orvosi Hetilap* essay. In fact, he incorporated major parts of it into his treatise. However, *Aetiology* was something more. It would serve as a vent, a cathartic for the rage that had been incubating within him for thirteen years, from the origin of his theory in 1847 until its publication in 1860.

Semmelweis began his diligent task, writing *Aetiology* in his spare time, in mid-1858. As if taking on that challenge was not enough, he accepted another time-consuming task—editing parts of a journal of obstetrics and gynecology. He worked at both simultaneously.[9] For a man already overworked, stealing hours from sleep and family time proved exhausting, yet he held out such great hope for the piece that he could not do otherwise. Finally, Semmelweis completed the work in October 1860, although its official publication date was 1861. With its 543 pages of meticulous detail and punctilious reasoning, *Aetiology* represented a Herculean effort. Still, Semmelweis scholars and biographers have described the author in consistently negative terms, calling him bellicose, angry, paranoid, eccentric, excitable, misanthropic, to name but a few. The treatise itself was wordy, rambling, disorganized, querulous, and burdened with excessive, aimless circumlocutions. No one has sought to argue with early translator Frank Murphy, who labeled the work as egotistic and lacking in any sense of progression. "We are conscious of signs of Semmelweis's mental aberration and feeling of persecution . . . the book itself discloses the underlying paranoia. If Semmelweis had only spent more time in clearly stating his views and less in argument his book would be twice as good and half as long!"[10]

Yet, on the positive side, Semmelweis presented his arguments in a rational, dialectic form, offering up various adversaries' assertions, before soundly destroying them with solid reasoning. At times he made liberal use of sarcasm to express contempt for his adversaries, whom he deemed professionally slothful or dishonest. He did not hesitate to use *ad hominem* attacks on his critics. While the macro-organization of the work may have been flawed, his points of argumentation on a more micro-level were generally solid, with cogent, measured steps of reasoning. Certain parts of the work are impassioned and even eloquent, offering a glimpse into the anguished ventilations of a persecuted man.

Semmelweis's propensity for composing elongated, detailed recitations and recapitulations of historical facts, combined with tedious, detailed statistical analyses of etiological argumentation, made the work difficult to read. If he received criticism from a colleague in the midst of his writing, he often interposed his retort to that colleague directly into the middle of his current exposition, giving the narrative both a sense of circumlocution and, as Murphy stated, little sense of forward progression. The man was so oblivious to standard literary conventions, that biographers described his manuscript as a copyeditor's nightmare.

According to Sinclair, when writing *Aetiology*, Semmelweis remained in a sustained state of excitement, frenetically producing fresh chapters and constantly repeating portions of his manuscript. Sinclair provides a confirmatory picture of Semmelweis's mental state through the eyes of Ignac Hirschler, oculist and then-chairman of the Medical Society of Pest. One day in 1860, Hirschler and Semmelweis happened to meet on the street, where Hirschler found Semmelweis to be "in a great state of excitement." Semmelweis led Hirschler back to his home, where he shared the Introduction with him. "He considered the work now complete; he had finished with the preface. . . . Yet it was not complete: Semmelweis was continually writing fresh chapters, all in a great hurry, constantly repeating portions without coordination, and hurrying the manuscript off to the printer without revision."[11]

Aetiology not only had an effect on the practitioners and biographers who read it, but it wrought even more remarkable physical effects on its author, as well. His frenzied state, sustained over a period exceeding two years, had wrought profound effects on Semmelweis, from both a physical as well as a mental standpoint.

As will become clear later, shortly before Semmelweis's death, an evaluating physician described a series of mental signs and symptoms from which Semmelweis suffered. According to German obstetrician and writer Georg Sillo-Seidl, that physician arranged those symptoms "to create a textbook picture of manic-depressive mental illness without actually stating this diagnosis." But in the 1860s, that ailment had yet to be recognized or delineated as a distinct disease. Even Sillo-Seidl, in his 1978 biography, made no assertions that Semmelweis suffered from manic-depressive psychosis.[12] In fact, he drew no more specific conclusions than did any other biographer concerning Semmelweis's chronic mental state.

If one views *Aetiology* in the context of a writer who had been under the scourge of severe mood swings for nearly a decade, the work, with its lack of coherent plotting, flight of ideas, bellicosity, grandiosity, and prolix, could be seen in a more specific light. Semmelweis's frenetic writing activity, plus the work product itself, provide evidence that he was in a sustained manic or hypomanic phase of a bipolar illness, evident since sometime between 1858 and 1860. His earlier overt eccentricities and autonomous mood swings suggest that he had been in the incipient stages of the disease even before 1858. In all likelihood, bipolar disease had been dominating his life, in varying degrees, for many years.

In Semmelweis's era, the diagnosis of manic-depressive illness was virtually nonexistent. Patients presenting with mental ailments were diagnosed as suffering from either mania, depression, or some other variant of mood dysfunction. The idea of manic-depressive illness as a single entity, mania and depression existing within the same person, was unheard of. In 1854, two Frenchmen working independently, J. P. Falret and Jules Baillarger, first posited the idea that mania and depression could possibly exist as a single entity within the same patient. Falret named the condition "circular insanity," while Baillarger called it "double insanity." Both names meant the same thing: the ailment was a single disease existing within a single patient, one phase of the illness cycling into the other in a never-ending state.[13] But it is doubtful that any patient presenting outside of France in 1865 with manifestations of manic-depressive illness would have been recognized as suffering from a distinct entity by any name. Medical journalism and the interchange of information in the nineteenth century, especially between countries speaking different languages, was a slow and uncertain process.

In fact, it was not until the 1890s that Munich psychiatrist Emil Kraepelin began to distinguish "circular insanity" from dementia praecox (schizophrenia). Through years of experience and data collection on mental patients, Kraepelin gave to the discipline of psychiatry the first tenable classification of manic-depressive illness in all of its nuanced forms. However, it was not until 1913 that he finally unified the two maladies, mania and depression, convincingly into one entity, a concept that, despite some recent challenges, still stands today. Kraepelin was also the first to point out that psychological stresses experienced on a daily basis were themselves powerful enough to precipitate episodes of mental aberration—a point of particular interest for the chronically stressed Semmelweis.[14]

In Semmelweis's personal life, the depressive aspect of the disease certainly dominated his persona, but that is the more typical face presented by manic-depressive illness. According to University of Colorado psychology professor David J. Miklowitz, patients typically suffer from cycles of depression that are three time longer in duration than are their manic phases.[15] Still, in Semmelweis's case his mental state, as reflected in his writings, was more consistent with mania, given his prolix, flight of ideas, certitude, humility juxtaposed with megalomania, punctilious reasoning, self-righteousness, irritability, and underlying angry tone.

According to Miklowitz, the more stressful the lives of bipolar patients are, the less stable, in general, will their clinical courses be. The mental states of individual patients are subject to both biologic and social rhythms. Some social influences, such as support from a loved one or other similarly soothing events, exert a positive effect on a patient's psyche. These influences exert an overall positive effect on one's clinical course. On the negative side are the influences that disrupt a patient's daily social rhythms, exerting, in turn, an overall deleterious effect on the patient's illness. Such events could be something as vague as traveling to a different time zone, a new romantic interest, or even the birth of a child.[16] Certainly Semmelweis had his problems with ongoing life stressors, all of which were negative except for his peaceful home life. It was at home with the family where he sought and apparently received comfort, sheltered from life's daily storms. The abundance of negative stressors, plus the fact that no definitive treatment existed for bipolar disease in the nineteenth century, makes it less than surprising that Semmelweis's problems worsened with time.

Whatever his mental state, when it came to writing *Aetiology*, Semmelweis did manage to organize it into seven parts, including Autobiographical Introduction, the Concept of Childbed Fever, Aetiology, short sections on Endemic Disease and Prophylaxis, plus two minor parts.[17] The earlier sections were a recapitulation of his transition from orthodoxy to heterodoxy, a history of his path to enlightenment. These earlier parts, although plagued by the aforementioned repetitions, were well reasoned and comparatively unemotional. In medical school, he, like all other students, had been indoctrinated, essentially force fed a diet of *Genius epidemicus* theory. It was only after gaining clinical experience and beginning his research effort that his own convictions concerning the manner in which diseases actually developed began to surface. Early in *Aetiology*, Semmelweis declared puerperal fever to be, "*without exception of a single case*," [italics his] a resorption fever.[18] Puerperal fever was a variety of pyemia, a blood poisoning, almost always introduced into the patient from the external environment. That single event, absorption of contaminant, was responsible for all the epidemics so feared by physicians and public alike. Once a practitioner recognized this fact of absorption, the disease was virtually 100 percent preventable—self-infection being the only exception to the rule. Degenerating animal-organic matter might already be residing within the patient as a result of degenerated lochia, blood, or retained placenta. With time that source could deteriorate into infection. Self-infection, which accounted for approximately 1 percent of cases, could not be prevented.

Sources of degenerating animal-organic matter were: the cadaver, regardless of gender, gravid or not; draining wounds of the living; and other infected patients, whether from a surgical or medical source. In Pest, the greatest source proved to be bed linens stained with lochia and blood, negligently reused for patients in the early stages of labor. Carrier: unlike cholera or smallpox, puerperal fever was not contagious through casual patient contact. Rather, it was conveyed to a new patient by a caretaker's examining finger, operating hand, bed clothes and linens, and other objects.[19] Site of infection: infection occurred when contaminated matter was introduced into the internal os (mouth) of the cervix, or upwards into the uterus, the site of placental implantation, or the fallopian tubes. Any part of the genital tract that was injured was capable of absorption. Time of infection: theoretically, one could become infected during any phase of pregnancy, if the cervical os was not closed. Practically, however, all cases occurred during labor as the examining finger encountered a dilated cervix. Infection rarely occurred during the expulsive phase. A dilated, patulous birth canal, early after labor, could even be infected by air itself, if the air was sufficiently contaminated with noxious effluvia.[20] With his reasoning so cogent, how could it have been that difficult for the practitioner to understand? That is, if he even bothered to read it.

Semmelweis claimed that his main aims in publishing *Aetiology* were not only to destroy the faulty reasoning of his critics, but to repudiate, in particular, the *Genius epidemicus* and cosmic-atmospheric-telluric theories. He began by describing puerperal fever as a "blood poisoning." While not epidemic or contagious in the usual sense, blood poisoning could be conveyed to others via the items and methods he had listed above. It could be conveyed from a sick parturient to a healthy pregnant woman only if the former produced decomposed material that was then conveyed to the healthy one. Semmelweis explained further that, "After death puerperal fever is conveyable from every cadaver of a puerpera to a healthy individual when the cadaver has reached the necessary degree of decomposition."[21] It was popular to name epidemic influences, cosmic-atmospheric-telluric conditions, wounded modesty, emotion, poor diet, and so forth as important in causing puerperal fever, yet no such forces played any significant role in its origin. Men could not control the weather. Therefore, if atmospheric mechanisms were the cause, the disease would be unpreventable. Such reasoning made men adopt a fatalistic, *laisser faire* attitude. The English enjoyed a lower mortality rate than did the Germans and the French. Yet all countries were subjected to the same atmospheric conditions. English rates were lower because they employed the chloride wash.[22]

Seasons, as such, had no influence on the incidence of puerperal fever. If seasonal variations had such a strong influence on the incidence of puerperal fever, why then did Boer, who enjoyed a constant 1 percent infection rate, see no variation with the seasons? Similarly, before Semmelweis's arrival at St. Rochus Hospital, the disease raged in the months of August and September, a time when it should have been, by epidemicists' reasoning, in its quiescent phase. All cases of puerperal fever were due to a single phenomenon—the resorption of decaying animal-organic matter. "As living proof of my doctrine," Semmelweis declared, "I decreased puerperal fever mortality rates in three different hospitals by utilizing my regimen."[23] Semmelweis concluded by stating, "The doctrine of epidemic puerperal fever explains something unknown [puerperal fever], by that which is also unknown."[24] That second "unknown," of course, was bacteria. But decades would ensue before the disease-causing role of bacteria would be recognized.

Semmelweis then included two shorter sections concerning endemic disease and prophylaxis. The first section, regarding self-infection, conveyed little new information, while the second was, in essence, a short primer on prevention. "Whoever practices this prophylaxis will experience the pleasure, not from time to time to lose every third or every fourth patient from puerperal fever, but perhaps to lose only one in four hundred."[25]

Semmelweis's last section, "Correspondence and Opinions in the Literature for and against My Doctrine," constituted the longest and most contentious part of *Aetiology*. Here, his anger and contempt towards his adversaries reached its full expression. His fury was fueled not only by the dishonesty and misrepresentations he had encountered over a dozen years, but, as well, by the failure of physicians to accept a simple truth—a blindness born of complacency. Were such obstetrical agnostics ever to experience that epiphany, the truth became nearly self-evident. Sadly, generations of professionals went forth, instead, into villages, where they spread infection as a consequence of their ignorance. Semmelweis's corrective efforts were spurred by their simple failure to learn a theory and apply it in a beneficent manner. "I think it would be criminal behaviour on my part," he wrote, "if I were longer to remain silent, and neglect producing unbiased, impartial, and complete evidence in favour of the practical extension of my Doctrine."[26]

Semmelweis believed that his message held such great potential for humanity that he began referring to it by the vainglorious term "eternally true doctrine," an assertion that further enabled his critics to label him at least egotistical, if not megalomaniacal. He was asking the medical world to surrender their long-held humoral theories in favor of some belief that a simple contaminant residing within decaying animal-organic matter was the sole cause of a disease that had not only plagued mankind for centuries, but the origin of which had proved insoluble to so many great minds. How could men, who were accustomed to thinking about disease causation in multifactorial terms, accept such a simplistic view?

Semmelweis devoted more than two hundred pages of this section to answering his critics. He had his supporters, such as Haller, Routh, Michaelis, and Tilanus, yet Semmelweis saved his energy for his illustrious adversaries, more than twenty in all. He directed most of his rage at his prime target, Wilhelm Scanzoni, who, by 1860, was considered Germany's foremost accoucheur. With Scanzoni's lack of understanding of puerperal fever, this died-in-the-wool epidemicist proved an easy target. In Scanzoni's mind, puerperal fever could be divided into two types: those with and those without blood disintegration. But, as he viewed the problem, epidemic influences clearly stood at the root of the disease. He admitted to having tried chloride washings in an 1848 Prague epidemic, only to find them ineffective. Semmelweis responded sarcastically, "I cannot deny my wonder at Scanzoni's penetrating sagacity in dispensing with chlorine washings as an experiment."[27] Semmelweis openly taunted his main target for being a miserable failure. When Scanzoni experienced unfavorable results after employing chloride washings for less than a six-month period, he hastily concluded that they had been of no importance.[28]

To Scanzoni's earlier charge that Skoda had never proved statistically in his addresses that puerperal fever could be characterized as a pyemia, Semmelweis countered: every case of puerperal fever is a case of pyemia, without exception. With his erroneous sense of pyemia, Scanzoni provided a "defective, entirely worthless classification of puerperal inflammations; for him the essence of childbed fever is *terra incognita*."[29] Semmelweis mocked Scanzoni's "mistake-ridden classification" of puerperal inflammations. He must have copied it from others "because the nature of puerperal fever is unknown to him."[30] Responding to Scanzoni's lamentation of how unfortunate it was that "our investigations of the atmospheric-terrestrial-cosmic factors have not, as yet, given us much positive understanding of these phenomena," Semmelweis replied, "Naturally, one cannot have much positive understanding of that which does not exist."[31]

Scanzoni, continuing his wrongheaded views on etiology, later asserted that "I myself fear nothing so much as when a patient is suddenly seized by great fear, anger or worry. . . I have observed many cases in which there is no doubt that such an emotional disturbance provided the essential cause of puerperal sickness."[32] Surrendering once again to sarcasm, Semmelweis observed that since "Scanzoni has so often shown himself to be a wretched observer," it is much more likely that "he or someone else infected the patient and that between the time of the infection and the outbreak of fever, emotional disturbances occurred." To Scanzoni's assertion that epidemics were miasmatic in origin, Semmelweis countered that the influence was found in decaying matter, not in some miasm. Scanzoni believed in miasms, yet "he utters not a syllable as to how one can prevent or destroy the miasma. This reflects Scanzoni's thoughtlessness in writing about things he does not understand."[33]

In yet another article, Scanzoni disputed Semmelweis's claim that cadaveric particles, adhering to examiners' hands, caused puerperal fever by contaminating the injured genitalia of those in labor.[34] Semmelweis derided Scanzoni, calling him an "epidemicist," hoping to brand him with the archaic image the term invoked.[35] Scanzoni's ideas of etiology did not withstand criticism. He was correct on a few minor facts, but "all the rest appears to be a mass of error and confusion." "No patients have died of childbed fever as a result of emotional disturbances, of mistakes in diet, or of puerperal miasma," Semmelweis declared, "because puerperal miasma does not exist as Scanzoni conceives it."[36]

Semmelweis had grown suspicious of Scanzoni's rosy claims regarding his six-year mortality rates in Wurzburg—rates even lower than Semmelweis had experienced after instituting chloride washings in Vienna. Dubious of his claim, Semmelweis challenged Scanzoni by throwing his own claims of etiology back in his face: "Herr Hofrath [esteemed professor], you must account to the world how it happened that for six years you had such a favorable state of health among the puerperae at the same institution in which Kiwisch had" such a high mortality rate.[37] "What have you done, Herr Hoffrath?" Semmelweis inquired. Had the puerperae "not had the composition of the blood peculiar to gravidae, which predisposes them to puerperal fever? Did the favorable *Genius epidemicus*, which in the Prague Lying-In-Hospital lasted only one month after the introduction of the chlorine washings, prevail in Wurzburg for six years? Was there no winter in Wurzburg for six years, which brought no cold damp days?" Among those Scanzoni cared for, Semmelweis demanded, "were there no women weak, badly nourished, exposed during pregnancy to privation and need, or living under the influence of depressing mental states?" Were these women "devoid of all sense of shame?" Semmelweis pressed on:

> Or were they not used as material for examination or observation? Do the Wurzburg men examine with greater delicacy of feeling? Have these puerperae committed no errors of diet? What have you done, Herr Hofrath, that the puerperal miasma cannot exert its murderous energy in the Wurzburg Lying-in Hospital?[38]
>
> Is Herr Hoffrath a more successful observer of my doctrine in private and my adversary only in public, since the time when he would not deny such infections in single cases? Have you, Herr Hoffrath, such an aversion to the truth, that you awarded a prize to Dr. Silberschmidt's work, although he suppressed the truth about your favorable results in Wurzburg. Or does the Herr Hoffrath live in the conviction that you shine only when surrounded by darkness?[39]
>
> You build your greatness, Herr Hoffrath, upon the stupe-

faction of those unfortunate parturients who will be ground down in death by those whom you have made stupid. Should even human justice remain inactive in the face of conduct fraught with such misfortune, Herr Hoffrath, you will not escape God's justice.[40]

Semmelweis's attack against Scanzoni continued for a total of 103 pages, until he must have felt, at least momentarily, purged of his rage.

For his next target, Semmelweis chose the celebrated polymath, Rudolf Virchow, professor of pathology at the University of Berlin, venerated father of cellular pathology, published archeologist, and liberal German parliamentarian. Despite having no direct clinical experience with puerperal fever, Virchow never hesitated to interject his opinion into the debate.[41] In fact, his august opinions proved to be a major impediment to the spread of Semmelweis's doctrine for decades. Virchow refused to accept Semmelweis's contention that pyemia, whether consequent to puerperal fever or to the disease that kills anatomists and surgeons wounded by contaminated knives, represented the same disease.

Virchow's public statement of 1856 stirred further resentment in Semmelweis: "For the occurrence of puerperal fever epidemics two conditions of interest are essential: the state of the weather and the occurrence of certain diseases simultaneously. . . . To the simultaneous diseases belong the acute exanthemata [rashes], the extensive spread of erysipelatous, croupous, putrid and purulent inflammations. The more poorly the uterus and neighboring vessels contract increases the chances of fibrin formation in blood. That plus a 'special nervous influence' leads to childbed fever."[42]

Semmelweis could agree with Virchow on one point. Puerperal fever often did occur concurrent with erysipelas or other diseases, but only because patients with such diseases were frequently cared for by the same practitioners who also treated pregnant women. If such caregivers were ignorant of the cause of puerperal fever, the two diseases would naturally wax and wane in a coordinated manner.[43] Only Virchow believed that thrombosis led to puerperal fever. Unfortunately, because of Virchow's position of authority, he made error seem credible to his followers:

By what right does Virchow lend the authority of his name to this declaration, the same Virchow, who indeed has not yet attacked my doctrine because he ignores it in his supreme vanity. My students, medical men, surgeons and 823 female students who have been trained by me as midwives for obstetrical practice in Hungary, who know better than Virchow why the great majority of puerperal epidemics occur in winter, who know better than Virchow what to do in order not to have concurrent puerperal fever, when patients with erysipelatous, croupous, ichorous, and purulent inflammations are committed to their care; who in their enlightenment as members of the Society of Obstetrics would laugh at Virchow, if he would lecture them on epidemic puerperal fever.[44]

As a highly respected international figure in medicine, Virchow was used to polite argumentation, if not totally deferential treatment. Semmelweis was accusing Virchow, the man who had published his celebrated work on cellular pathology in 1847, of being a "bad observer." Semmelweis's sarcasm, his belittling of this sage, was shocking, but, in his rage, Semmelweis deferred to no one.

The ever resolute Virchow repeated his opinions at the obstetrical meeting in Berlin's Charité Hospital in 1858. In fact, his open attacks on Semmelweis continued until as late as 1864.

Semmelweis next aimed his arrow at Carl Braun. He was concerned that Braun's opinion might bear greater weight than some of his other critics, since the two men shared a common origin in Vienna's Division I. They might, therefore, have similar insights. Feeling duty-bound to crush the man, Semmelweis devoted over forty pages refuting Braun's misconceptions. As Semmelweis observed, Braun fortunately had made his task easy since he so frequently "says silly things."[45] Braun's opposition to the eternally true etiology came not from a conviction that the theory was untrue, but rather from his ignorance of the most important precepts of the theory and, as well, from his ill will. "Does it not point to ill will, if Carl Braun states my propositions in very many places, and then opposes the same propositions in the clinic for 12 papers and in his text-book for 4 papers?"[46] As evidence, Semmelweis cited Braun's own belief, expressed in his *Clinic for Obstetrics and Gynecology*: since puerperal fever or pyemia is engendered by the inoculation of, among other things, cadaveric poison, "it is therefore the strict duty of the physician to see to the rigid isolation of healthy puerperae from those ill from zymotic disease . . . and never to examine or operate on a gravida, parturient or puerpera, if an assistant had any contact a short time before with cadaveric particles or septic exudates."[47] In the same book, Braun admonished every clinician to perform their clinical examinations "in the earliest morning hours before there is any sort of contact with cadavers." Given such statements, Semmelweis wondered, "Can Carl Braun oppose me with the conviction that my doctrine is false?"[48]

So opposed to chloride washings was Braun that he abandoned them early in his Division I tenure. He advised his students to instead, refrain from examining patients if, after washing with soap and water, their hands still gave off a cadaveric odor. In *Aetiology* Semmelweis waded through the minutia of his own departmental statistics, lucidly pointing out Braun's mistaken position on the washings, plus his failure to teach the chloride regimen to the one hundred fifty to two hundred students he trained annually. "And what harm will these students, so badly taught by Carl Braun, do out in practice?" They will go out into the public as trained infectors. Semmelweis also cited the case of Gustav Braun, Carl's brother and successor in Division I, who suffered a "ghastly accomplishment": 717 "unnecessary" deaths, for the same reasons.[49]

Braun had expressed strong disagreement with Semmelweis's 1847 announcement that cadaveric particles were the "exclusive cause" of puerperal fever. He was even more amazed when "Semmelweis found a supporter in this matter in Professor Skoda!!"[50] Braun's assertion forced Semmelweis to respond in *Aetiology*, using the expanded term "decomposed organic matter" rather than cadaveric particles. He patiently reiterated the steps involved in the development of puerperal fever once the caregiver becomes contaminated. Semmelweis had to wonder about Braun. If he does not believe that the cadaver is the source of infection, "why then does he enjoin his students with utmost conscientiousness not to examine parturients, if on the same day they have had contact with a cadaver? It is curious that Braun has no trouble attacking the theory while at the same time he exercises precautions against infection. He practices antisepsis himself."[51] By denying something on one hand, yet showing it respect on the other, Braun perpetuated a falsehood. "C. Braun reproaches me because I depend on the past, and draw therefrom very bold conclusions," Semmelweis contended, "I reproach C. Braun because he depends mostly on the present and draws therefrom false conclusions."[52]

Semmelweis devoted many pages defending his doctrine against Braun in a point/counterpoint fashion. He enumerated some of his different propositions with which Braun strongly disagreed, including the lack of influence the season of the year had on puerperal fever, the importance of ichorous fluids in disease causation, and the inexplicably low incidence of puerperal fever in conditions such as street births, as well as premature and precipitous deliveries, to mention but a few. He destroyed Braun's arguments sequentially using simple logic buttressed by the tables of statistics that he had compiled through his years of research.[53]

Before dispensing with his adversary completely, Semmelweis next addressed Braun's list of thirty causes of puerperal fever as compiled in his *Clinic for Obstetrics and Gynecology*– the same piece that listed cadaveric infection as number twenty-eight. Semmelweis freely admitted that ten out of the thirty "causes" could be legitimate, such as 10) the birth act itself; 14) protracted labor; 21) operative intervention; and, of course, 28) cadaveric infection, among several others. The other twenty so-called causes, such as miasmatic air, emotional stress, embarrassment, and the like were each irrelevant. They were "either not causes of childbed fever, or even if they are . . . they are such only because through these irrelevant conditions in the lying-in-hospitals a decomposed matter is introduced into a patient from without."[54] After methodically destroying each of Braun's other "causes" with punctilious reasoning and argumentation, Semmelweis concluded that: "To Carl Braun, childbed fever is a zymotic disease of an acute character, which in the presence of a strong predisposition in the individual can engender decomposed animal matter by a general noxiousness, such as violent emotion, chilling, etc., as a rule by particular influences, miasma, contagion, whereby the extraneous characteristics work as a ferment and set up fermentation by contact with the blood mass."[55] It becomes obvious to the reader that Carl Braun: "The same Carl Braun, who so brilliantly attached [sic] the hypothesis of cadaveric infection based upon conjecture and lacking every direct proof, who to the satisfaction of every true friend of humanity has so triumphantly robbed the epidemic influences of their unlimited strength; the same Carl Braun allots indeed the decomposed animal, but not the epidemic influences a place in the concept of puerperal fever. O logic! O logic! We give therefore our Vienna colleague, while we bid him farewell, the cogent advice; not to neglect to take some semesters of logic as soon as possible, in case he should feel the need to take up the noble calling of battling for the epidemic death of purperae [sic]."[56]

Semmelweis had one other point of contention with Braun that needed to be settled. Braun had previously declared that Semmelweis had announced his theory of cadaveric infection more than five years ago, yet, "Nowhere in the literature do we find any acknowledgement of the credibility of the infection-theory in its practical application."[57] Semmelweis countered with the obvious. During his years in Vienna, he had proved that his doctrine was "an eternally true fact." Furthermore: "What is true in Vienna, is true for the whole world, and if the truth, which could be established in Vienna, cannot be established elsewhere, then the truth does not thereby become a falsehood, but anyone who could not establish the truth has proven his own incompetency."[58]

After dispensing with Braun, *Aetiology* ended, but Semmelweis did add a brief epilogue. Writing this polemic had not been occasioned by some "quarrelsome disposition." It had, rather, been his sacred duty. Claiming that he was able to discern optimism through his melancholic haze, Semmelweis sensed a happy future in which the scourge of puerperal fever would finally be conquered. Lying-in hospitals the world over would find themselves in that preferable state of experiencing only those inevitable cases of auto-infection.[59]

Reaction to *Aetiology*

When Semmelweis finally saw *Aetiology* come off the press in October 1860, he was buoyant. He proudly sent courtesy copies to many medical societies and influential obstetricians throughout Europe, anxiously hoping that his treatise would prove to be a major turning point in physicians' attitudes. While waiting, he buried himself in his practice and university duties. One would think that his two main targets, Scanzoni and Braun, would have prepared vigorous defenses, but such was not the case. Both merely ignored Semmelweis's charges. Most of the early comments came from individual obstetricians. A few of the more enlightened respondents expressed favorable opinions. Robert Froriep, editor of the *Notizen*, stated that the "author's discovery is one of the most significant events in modern medicine, so we wish to present it to our readers in a special number, discussing the essential points herewith."[1] Another, Professor Kugelmann of Hanover, replied, "Permit me . . . to express the holy joy with which I studied your work. . . . I felt myself compelled to declare: This man is a second Jenner; may his services receive a similar recognition and his efforts bring him the enjoyment of a similar satisfaction." Kugelmann, who was in possession of an autographed copy of Jenner's pioneering work, offered it to Semmelweis "as a mark of my unlimited respect." In a follow-up letter he stated prophetically, "It has been vouchsafed to very few to confer great and permanent benefits upon mankind, and with few exceptions the world has crucified and burned its benefactors. . . . I hope you will not grow weary in the honourable fight which still remains before you."[2] But it was not to be.

French accoucheur C. S. F. Credé wrote a review of *Aetiology*, in which he admitted that the author and his chloride regimen had obvious merit. However, he, like some of his colleagues, was concerned that other unknown factors lay behind the etiology of childbed fever. "The book is worth studying by every expert, yet it does not serve the cause to call everybody who does not agree ignorant or even a murderer."[3]

Old adversary Franz Zipfl continued to express strong disagreement with Semmelweis, stating that puerperal fever was obviously caused by epidemic influences.[4] Joseph Spaeth dismissed the work as so much old news. Such facts had been known for fourteen years. Spaeth had just published an article in March 1861 asserting that some real serious contributions to puerperal fever had been made when Martin, Wagner, and others elucidated "the connection between salpingitis [tubal infection]and peritonitis."[5]

Aetiology fared little better with the medical press. Most editorials limited their commentaries on the work to a few brief, forgettable lines, leaving the author troubled by their lack of respect. How could such a major achievement elicit so little reaction? He began having major doubts that his Herculean effort in writing *Aetiology* would ever have any widespread, meaningful impact. Was the general obstetrical community, still clinging to Old School attitudes, intellectually incapable of understanding his theory? Or had they, as some suggested, simply made an overt decision to ignore it based upon some sort of chauvinistic attitude? Whatever their reasons, the general inaction of the press and the obstetrical community wounded Semmelweis deeply. His early hope slowly changed to disappointment, which turned to anger. The bitter blows left him ever more desperate for a triumph.

Faithful friend and confidant Markusovsky was troubled enough by the remarks of Semmelweis's critics to come to his aid in 1861. In fact, Marko, during Semmelweis's career, functioned in much the same manner as Thomas H. Huxley did with Charles Darwin. Like Semmelweis, the genial Darwin expressed an innate aversion to all forms of contention and polemic. Huxley, always anxious for a fight, consistently rose up in the scientist's defense, earning him the moniker "Darwin's Bulldog." Marko felt a similar allegiance to Semmelweis. Writing a review of *Aetiology* in his *Medical Weekly*, he stated, "As I perused it and considered its effect on myself, I must confess that it is more than a scientific book or treatise, though each of its theories rests on pathological research, on clinical observation and statistical data, and its rationation is on the highest methodological level." Since the value of the theory was beyond question, Marko continued:

> It is quite absurd that we should still hear *ex cathedra* theories and aetiologies. It is preposterous that when counting for the causation of puerperal fever medical students should still speak of cold and heat, hunger and gluttony, hyperinosis and uremia, plethora and hydremia, congestion and inopexia, activity and inertia, sorrow and outraged modesty, etc., etc. . . . Instead of denying the above causes, the German and French obstetricians have even added new items to the list. The *genius endemicus* and *epidemicus* have not been ousted from the field of childbed fever; on the contrary, the greatest medical authorities have risen in their favour in the Paris academies, and, in spite of the discovery of Semmelweis, they still prevail in the lying-in hospitals in Vienna. Ever since the days of Boer, unbiased, sober experience cannot be tolerated there.[6]

Then there was the criticism of August Briesky, a member of the Prague School. Many obstetricians considered his opinion to be noteworthy since he represented a cross section of the entire German establishment. Being as biased against Semmelweis as was his old colleague Scanzoni, Briesky attempted to diminish Semmelweis with derision, referring to him as the "Apostle of Cadaveric Infection." As for *Aetiology*, it was naive, "the Koran of a puerperal creed which he preaches with a fanatical zeal and enters into battle with threatenings of fire and sword for the unbelievers."[7] Briesky concluded his criticism by charging that Semmelweis had never identified any particle unique to decaying matter that might have led him to the derivation of his theory. "There is the 'something' which is yet unknown in the etiology and has still to be discovered."[8]

Markusovsky again came to the rescue of his reticent friend with yet another *Medical Weekly* article, "Some Voices against the Semmelweis Doctrine Concerning the Aetiology of Puerperal Fever."

Marko wisely sensed that most accoucheurs did not seem to understand the concept of "single and necessary" in the context of disease
causation. In the case of puerperal fever, that "single and necessary"
factor was some as yet unexplained and undiscovered particle in decomposing animal-organic matter.

Referring to Briesky, Marko admitted that perhaps additional evidence as to the cause of the disease might yet be gathered. He pointed out how Semmelweis, at this time, remained more concerned
about preventing the disease, since countless lives were being lost
needlessly. Semmelweis himself did not consider his theory to be
cast in stone. Even though one might best consider it a work in
progress, few maladies in medical science had been better elucidated than childbed fever. Certainly more information was needed concerning the chemical and histological nature of the organic
matter, for example, how it was broken down and absorbed in the
body. Even more intriguingly, why in identical circumstances did
full blown disease occur in one patient and not in another? These
enigmas must be elucidated, yet: "Are we to draw the conclusion
that, because the new doctrine has not as yet been explained in every detail, it is therefore false, and that the ancient definiteness of
epidemic darkness is to be preferred? . . . The rule of logic stipulates
in all observations that if we are able to attribute a phenomenon to
a certain source, we should look for this cause in every individual
case, or else we lose grip completely and lose ourselves in the darkness of arbitrary supposition."[9] Of course, when it came to medical
theories of disease causation, arbitrary supposition was precisely
what physicians had been indulging in for millennia.

Unfortunately, Marko's thoughtful defense of Semmelweis, written exclusively in Hungarian, exerted little impact in silencing critics or creating converts. His article languished in relative obscurity
until biographer, Jakab Bruck, impressed by its sagacity, translated
it into German in 1887, much too late to exert any polemical effect
on Semmelweis's behalf.

Briesky was hardly the last to utter intolerant remarks against
Semmelweis. Professor Karl Hecker of Munich must have given
Semmelweis a profound sense of hopelessness with his blatant display of ignorance. Rejecting Semmelweis's doctrine outright, he
called it "one sided, narrow and erroneous." While reporting on an

epidemic within his own hospital, Hecker pointed to an enigma. His private obstetrical service had a "morbidity" of 4.9 percent, while his public clinic suffered at a rate of 16.3 percent. Demonstrating his impressive ignorance of the literature, Hecker charged that Semmelweis and his theory had never adequately explained two different phenomena: how was it that patients became sick in rows? Furthermore, why did newborns of mothers stricken with puerperal fever die just like their mothers? It was obvious from Hecker's clueless comments that he had either never read or had not comprehended *Aetiology*, nor was he familiar with Bednar's 1852 monograph concerning the deaths of such newborns. Hecker's report did, however, result in one positive response. It spurred Semmelweis to formally counter the man's nescience. In a June1862 letter to the editors of the *Medical Times and Gazette*, Semmelweis patiently restated his theory just as he had done so many times before.[10]

Several other adversaries, better known to Semmelweis, continued to utter erroneous facts in their critique of the theory. In early October 1860, Vienna's lying-in hospital suffered a flare up of puerperal fever, both in Division II, under the leadership of Franz Zipfl, and in Division I, headed by Carl Braun. Semmelweis, in comparison, had not experienced a single infection in his Budapest practice for the entire year 1860–1861. Directors of Vienna's hospital requested formal reports from both men explaining the reasons behind the high infection rate. Zipfl, having learned nothing since his 1850 debate with Semmelweis, blamed "unknown epidemic influences." "There can be no doubt of the existence here of a miasma, or rather of a contagium generating itself within the limits of the institution," he contended.[11] The 113 infections and 48 deaths in Braun's clinic generated much debate among hospital staff, prompting one staff member to suggest that perhaps the freshly published *Aetiology*, available for study that very month, could yield some answers to their conundrum. But Braun contended that no rational explanation for the infections existed. Hoping to deflect some of the blame, Braun asserted that, at the inception of the epidemic, one out of ten patients admitted was already in a "high state of fever." Clearly they were infected prior to entering the hospital. Braun's measures included discontinuing all student operations on cadavers. Declaring that the chloride regimen had been deemed worthless as

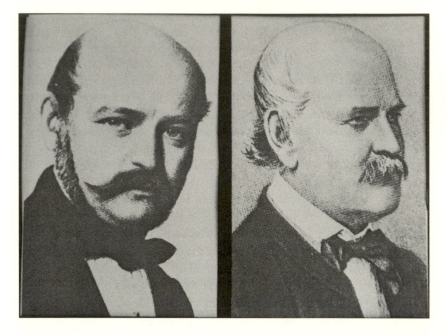

Figure 21. Contrasting images of Semmelweis illustrate the obvious physical effects associated with his literary effort. He is seen on the left in 1857, age thirty-nine, as he began his writing campaign. On the right is a photo taken a mere three years later, upon completion of *Aetiology*. He appears at least two decades older than his stated age of forty-two.

far back as 1854–1855, he instituted a similar routine but using a different chemical—permanganate of potash. Despite such measures, out of 253 admissions, 48 patients contracted puerperal fever in the first two weeks of November.[12]

Like the slow, erosive drip of water on stone, the illogical refutations of the *Lehre* and incessant attacks by the likes of Briesky, Hecker, Virchow, and others upon the man who had devoted his entire existence to the study of puerperal fever continued to exert their deleterious effects upon Semmelweis's psyche. His prolonged struggle against this impenetrable wall of complacency, his multiple disappointments, and the obvious deceitfulness of his many critics took their toll. His underlying moods became ever darker. Minor provocations, especially if they involved his theory, could send him into fits of rage. His angst manifested itself physically as well. For those who worked around him on a daily basis, the changes might have been insidious enough that they could have gone unnoticed. But if one compares a photograph taken in 1857, when he was thirty-nine, with one taken in 1860, at the conclusion of writing *Aetiology*, the preternatural changes are striking. In the latter photo he appears at least two decades older than his actual age of forty-two.[13]

Despite such deep anxiety, Semmelweis continued to draw strength from his enduring belief that "fate had selected him to be the champion of justice." In writing *Aetiology*, he had laid out all aspects of his theory and answered his critics as completely as possible. Still holding some sliver of hope for a watershed moment, he was determined to allow just a little more time.[14] Perhaps the obstetricians of Europe needed a little more time to accept it.

Open Letters

Semmelweis waited one long year for some major confirmatory statement on *Aetiology* before he sadly concluded that it would never come. Despite his mental fatigue and innumerable disappointments, the man with the iron will still refused to succumb to the implacable forces set against him. As he struggled to keep his pent-up emotions in check, Semmelweis made a decision. Seeing it as his sacred duty, he would launch a second general offensive. "I shall take consolation in the conviction that my action is not an end but a means . . . ," he explained, "to force many physicians to retrace their steps to the path of truth they have deviated from, at the expense of mankind, misled by the siren-voices of my enemies."[1]

His upcoming effort, *Open Letters*, would evolve into an even more intense expression of his rage towards those who refused to accept his *Lehre*—in particular, those esteemed professors in the major European universities. They needed to be exposed for their antediluvian views and their murderous ways. While such a sentiment may have been true, Semmelweis himself was approaching his writing effort from an even more extreme position, mentally. In his 1904 *Book of Obstetrics*, Tivadar Kezmarsky, Semmelweis's eventual successor in Budapest, related how Semmelweis had become constantly preoccupied with his theory. When he realized that his prolonged quest in spreading the word was a losing cause, the pace of his mental decline purportedly increased.[2] "He was duly irascible faced with the obstinate disregard of his documented doctrine," Kezmarsky reported, "despairing in the conviction that nevertheless it was his sacred duty to propagate his teachings, even with pen dipped in gall, with excruciating weapons, defying his opponents in his *Open Letters*, accusing them and stamping them before the world of science."[3]

Even Waldheim, one of Semmelweis's earliest biographers, who declared his subject to be eccentric as far back as 1850, believed him to be overtly mentally ill at least as early as 1859.[4] Maria, Semmelweis's wife, gives further evidence concerning distinct changes occurring at that time. In an October 1906 interview, forty years after the fact, she revealed that her husband had suffered from obvious "nervous complaints" since 1861.[5] Istvan Benedek, biographer and Budapest psychiatrist, while being struck by Semmelweis's early physical "senescence," claimed that he was, as well, absent-minded, loquacious, consumed his food "conspicuously," burst into tears without reason, and was predisposed to fits of anger. Benedek concluded, "The above list, together with the already mentioned premature ageing (*senium praecox*) unequivocally and unquestionably show that Semmelweis suffered from some sort of chronic disorder in the mental system, most probably progressive paralysis."[6] Although there is little to support Benedek's claim of progressive paralysis (tertiary or neurosyphilis), as will be discussed later, Semmelweis was clearly worsening mentally.

Benedek gave perhaps the best description of Semmelweis's persona and his deteriorating mental state when, between 1862 and 1863, his mood swings had progressed to even darker places with more prolonged and distinct extremes of depression. Benedek, while appearing to contradict himself by claiming that Semmelweis did not suffer from a "constitutional mental disturbance," went on to state that:

His whole life shows it clearly that he was a psychopathic personality. He was tormented, irritable, hot tempered, monomaniacally clinging to his own sphere of thought, in consequence quarrelsome even with his friends, rash in his judgement [*sic*] on those who looked unfavourably upon his hypothesis, often coarse. His psychopathic behavior was striking, especially in the sixties, when he worked himself up into a frenzy about debating. Markusovsky notes about that period that his manners became unbearable even within the circle of his friends: they dreaded his passionate strom [excitement] in defending his assertions, reviling his supposed or real opponents, and ranging

even his best-wishers among his enemies. In his polemical essays he did not refrain himself from using the most extreme
personal insults, which in many cases were even not justified;
he could not weigh his words. He preached his doctrine as
"solely true," "true forever," and in order to prove it he fell
into constant repetition.[7]

Obstetrician and writer Alfred Hegar gives confirmatory evidence: "His [Semmelweis's] mental irritability had increased ever
since he had become involved in extensive literary commitment.
Inducement to write was also caused by chronic impulses, and his
great book was followed, in quick succession, by his controversial
letters addressed to professors Siebold, Scanzoni, Spaeth, and the
last one addressed to all the professors of obstetrics. Unrestrained
argumentation, the use of strong language, words of abuse and constant repetition—all these point to the abnormal activity of psychic
factors. . . . His excited state of mind and uncompromising humour
were followed by intermittent periods of depression and melancholia. . . . The disease had developed very slowly, and neither his family nor his friends had seen the initial menace."[8]

But as early as 1862, Maria, Marko, Hirsch, and other friends
had noted similarly disturbing changes that would suggest bipolar
disease to the modern reader. They described him as "moody and
misanthropic," with periods of mental expansiveness followed by
"extreme depression."[9] In that same 1906 interview, Maria identified her husband's breaking point. As he began writing his momentous book, she explained, "it was then that persistent persecution
unhinged his mind."[10] While some who observed his mercurial behavior and darker moods described him merely as eccentric or misanthropic, as more of his signature confrontations played out before
colleagues and hospital personnel, whispers of "chronic insanity"
began floating ever more frequently throughout the hallways.[11]

Two Open Letters

It was no accident that the voice expressed by Semmelweis in Open
Letters was even stronger than that in Aetiology. Dealing over the
years with passive aggressive, if not overtly resistant, hospital per-

sonnel, whatever respect he might have had for them had dwindled to nothing. While engaging in spirited disagreements with colleagues or hospital personnel, reacting with anger and contempt toward his adversaries had become his *modus operandi*. Brushing aside all thoughts of collegiality, he was completely indifferent to any feelings or thoughts of others—what adversaries might think of him. He consciously maintained that same attitude as he wrote *Open Letters*, displaying no concern about the niceties of rhetorical etiquette. He took special aim at his adversaries' habit of spreading erroneous facts regarding his theory. For *Open Letters*, his targets were Joseph Spaeth, professor of obstetrics at Vienna's Joseph Academy, and his old favorite, Professor Scanzoni of Wurzburg.

Semmelweis had not forgotten Spaeth's 1861 essay in which he had repeated the aforementioned praise for the "discovery" made by Anselm Martin and colleagues. Martin observed that salpingitis (infection of the fallopian tubes) was, in effect, the cause of peritonitis, as though the entire process arose *de novo* within the fallopian tubes. Semmelweis painstakingly regurgitated his same old riff: puerperal fever was, without exception, an absorption fever, caused by decomposed animal-organic matter. As that contaminant was absorbed into the body, a disintegration of the blood resulted that, in turn, caused a spreading of a variable number of exudates throughout the body. Making the point that disintegrating blood was the common denominator, he continued: "My book, *Aetiology*, appeared in October 1860. In the 1861 *Medical Yearbook*, you stated that Prof. Martin, and others . . . 'have made a remarkable contribution to the understanding of the true postpartum diseases by determining the relationship of salpingitis to peritonitis.' It is erroneous to say that salpingitis develops as a result of disintegration of the blood. One does not get meningitis by direct connection of the tubes to the meninges, but rather by disintegration of the blood that flows to the nervous system."[12]

Spaeth, who had studied under Semmelweis just after his historic discovery, should have known better than to make such a statement. Directing his remarks at the professor, Semmelweis continued, "I believe that your mind had not been sufficiently lighted by the puerperal sun, which rose in Vienna in 1847, however close to you it shone . . . thousands and thousands of lying-in women and newborn infants who might have been saved have lost their lives since 1847." Semmelweis, wondering if Spaeth had perhaps forgotten his experience in Vienna, reminded him what had occurred in the Vienna clinic between January 1847 and December 1858—a time when Spaeth had practiced there. In that decade, after Semmelweis exited Vienna, 1,924 women in the two divisions died unnecessarily from puerperal fever.[13]

> In this massacre, you, Herr Professor, have participated. There is no other course open for me except to keep watch and every man who dares spread dangerous errors regarding puerperal fever will find in me an active opponent: This murder must cease, and in order that the murder ceases, I will keep watch, and anyone who dares to propagate dangerous errors about Childbed Fever will find in me an eager adversary. In order to put an end to these murders, I have no resort but to mercilessly expose my adversaries, and no one whose heart is in the right place will criticize me for seizing this expedient.[14]

Semmelweis's letter to Wilhelm Scanzoni, professor of obstetrics at Wurzburg, was also written in 1861. In *Aetiology*, Semmelweis had earlier declared how he would relentlessly oppose anyone who spread errors about puerperal fever. In this letter to Scanzoni, Semmelweis expressed his continuing pique concerning Otto Franque's article in which he asserted that the 1859 Wurzburg epidemic was due to the *Genius epidemicus*.[15] Stating that he had no argument with Franque, who innocently adopted his superior's delusions and errors, Semmelweis declared, "my business is with you alone."[16] Semmelweis rejected Scanzoni's assertion that Wurzburg's epidemic was due to certain epidemic and atmospheric influences: "It is rather due to all who practice in Wurzburg, ignorant of how puerperal fever is prevented . . . and this ignorance is the fault of the Professors of Obstetrics from whom the practicing physicians learned obstetrics. And in this regard, you have, Herr Hofrath, sent out a significant contingent of unwitting murderers into Germany."[17]

Semmelweis claimed that in *Aetiology* he had proved with mathematical accuracy that atmospheric influences have never been operant in the causation of puerperal fever. The disease had always been transmitted through the ignorance of physicians and nurses, who caused high mortality among lying-in women. He then informed Scanzoni that, once the true cause of the disease was recognized by the physician, all the phenomena of childbed fever could be readily explained: "The greatest service rendered by it [accepting the theory] is that it teaches how the unhappiness wrought by the disease can be prevented with certainty and that it prescribes to the practitioner a recognized active method of prophylaxis. Your teaching, on the other hand, puts upon the practitioner the stamp of the Turk who, in fatalistic passive resignation, permits the disaster to overwhelm his lying-in patients."[18]

Semmelweis informed Scanzoni that he had devoted 103 pages in *Aetiology* to refuting his "errors and deceptions." He then proposed a challenge to his favorite target. If Scanzoni disagreed with the reasoning behind the *Lehre*, declare it in an open address: "If you regard my doctrine to be true, I hereby challenge you to declare it publicly, without reservation, not for my own satisfaction, but in order that your pupils, who outside of the Lying-In-Hospitals furnish you with the corpses for the substantiation of your doctrine, may be led to the truth. Should you, however, Herr Hofrath, without having disproved my doctrine continue to train your pupils in the doctrine of Epidemic Childbed Fever, I declare before God and the world that you are a murderer and the 'History of Childbed Fever' would not be unjust to you if it memorialized you as a medical Nero."[19]

Semmelweis was not yet through with his letter-writing campaign. In July 1861, he composed two more, one, yet again, to Scanzoni, his most contemptuous adversary, and the other to the highly regarded professor of obstetrics in Gottingen, Hofrath Eduard Siebold. While Semmelweis offered little new information in these letters, each gives further insight into his increasing exasperation with the complacent ignorance of establishment physicians and their failure to recognize the truth.

Semmelweis's second letter to Scanzoni was written in response to an article by Scanzoni protégé Otto Franque regarding the Wurzburg epidemic of 1860. Predictably, Scanzoni considered the cause of the epidemic to be atmospheric influences, rather than decomposed animal-organic matter. After urging Scanzoni to give his *Lehre* due consideration, Semmelweis apparently gave up, declaring, "You have demonstrated, Herr Hofrath, that in a new hospital like yours provided with the most modern furnishings and appliances, a good deal of homicide can be committed, where the required talent exists."[20]

Semmelweis and the "kindly and warm-hearted" Siebold, his next target, had been friends since the latter had visited Semmelweis both in the early years of Vienna and, later, in Budapest.[21] Their relationship had been cordial until 1861, when Siebold, in his *History of Obstetrics*, attacked Semmelweis's doctrine. Siebold, making the same mistake propagated by Skoda, believed that Semmelweis considered cadaveric particles to be the sole and universal cause of puerperal fever. While he gave Semmelweis his due regarding the practical value of prevention, he believed that, "It is going too far to maintain that this is the only cause of puerperal fever, and thus to explain its frequent occurrence and the malignant character, and the epidemic incidence and extension of the malady in lying-in institutions."[22]

Semmelweis, cautiously trying to honor their prior friendship, recalled with pleasure the time they had spent together in Vienna—a time in which the Division I had ceased to be a "state-supported murder-den" due exclusively to Semmelweis's regimen. But now, "Herr Hofrath has made himself responsible for the diffusion of error regarding puerperal fever."[23] Although Semmelweis admitted to sharing a pleasant time in Pest, now he was duty bound to express his disappointment in Siebold for making the same mistake as others regarding cadaveric infection. "That amounts to willful misrepresentation of my teaching or want of the ability to understand it," Semmelweis stated. He then charitably characterized Siebold as one who would not tolerate the massacre of pregnant women if only he knew the facts: "I beg you, Herr Hofrath, to acquire an intimate knowledge of the truth as it is set forth in my book, so that in accordance with your kind disposition, you will be able to find support for new opinions in the bright faces of your lying-in patients and in an empty mortuary."[24]

Becoming more emotional as he wrote, Semmelweis's tone changed. "You have read my book with so little understanding that you still find something enigmatic in puerperal fever," he contended, "whilst to those who have grasped the meaning of my teaching everything about puerperal fever is as clear as sunlight."[25]

Declaring his earnestness to rid the world of puerperal fever, Semmelweis put forth a "noble proposal" to Siebold: arrange a meeting of German obstetricians in August or September to debate the question of etiology. He avowed, "I am determined to stay there until I have succeeded in converting all participants to my opinion. Herr Hofrath, the groaning of the dying puerperae is stifling the voice of my heart while I am writing."[26] Siebold responded by stating, "I do not wish to bear a grudge to my friend Semmelweis, who wants to scorch me with the rays of the very puerperal sun . . . which has risen over him, for the simple reason that I am not ready to share his views of puerperal fever unconditionally."[27]

In September 1861, Siebold did attend a meeting of the German Society for the Advancement of Natural and Medical Science in Speyer but, sadly, Semmelweis had been neither invited nor even informed of the meeting. *Aetiology* and its author were reportedly much discussed—all in the negative with but one exception. Wilhelm Lange of Heidelberg reported on his own stellar success at decreasing mortality rates merely by adopting Semmelweis's *Lehre*.[28] But the views of the majority of attendees, including the likes of Virchow, Siebold, and known Semmelweis critic Hecker, were much more in concurrence with the opinion expressed by J. W. Betschler of Breslau. Betschler claimed that each variety of puerperal fever had its own specific etiology. The ill-read Hecker averred that the infection theory alone could not explain all the epidemics of puerperal fever.

When Semmelweis read of the Speyer gathering and the archaic opinions expressed in the proceedings, it aroused an even greater bitterness and indignation in him. What was the difference between this German colloquium and the French Academy meeting of 1858? Each gave voice to nearly as many theories as there were speakers. All attendees were adrift in a sea of ignorance, having learned nothing over the preceding three years. Unfortunately, Semmelweis could not even vent his frustrations to Siebold, who had died unexpectedly in October 1861, a mere month after the Speyer meeting. Marko was similarly incensed by the Speyer members' rebuff of Semmelweis. In 1862, he wrote in the *Medical Weekly* concerning *Open Letters*: "The author is delivering a smashing blow to his opponents in the question of puerperal fever, proving by infallible statistics and multiple arguments the truth of his theory. The victory of a good cause may be retarded, especially when delusions have

to be defeated, but the final triumph is assured. We feel confident
that the time will come when our author will be given full satisfaction, which cannot be anything else but the complete recognition
of his doctrine."[29] But, unsurprisingly, Semmelweis realized little
in terms of gratification from his publishing of *Open Letters*. No
sudden transformation in obstetrical attitudes or care came about as
a result of his latest efforts.

Letters to All Professors

Still enraged by his being shunned at the Speyer meeting and obsessed by the ignorant epidemicist theories Continental professors
fed to their students of obstetrics, Semmelweis decided to aim his
next letter at the source—all professors of midwifery in Europe. In
May 1862, he published what would be his last formal missive, *Open
Letters to All the Professors of Midwifery*. Nearly two years had
elapsed since publication of *Aetiology*, certainly a sufficient amount
of time for responsible obstetricians to have familiarized themselves
with its contents. In his new *Open Letters to All the Professors of
Midwifery*, an even more sober entreaty, Semmelweis offered little
new of a factual nature, essentially repeating what he had already
asserted in *Aetiology*. Given the complacency of his target audience,
however, that hardly seemed inappropriate. Semmelweis gave his
reason for writing: "There is no other course open to me but to put
an end to the murderous practices of my adversaries by exposing
them most ruthlessly: nobody with a feeling heart will take it amiss
but will understand that there is no other course open to me."[30]

The publisher's introductory remarks asserted that Semmelweis
would prove by "infallible statistics and multiple arguments" the
veracity of his *Lehre*. "We feel confident that the time will come
when our author will be given full satisfaction, which cannot be
anything else but the complete recognition of his doctrine," the
comments maintained.[31] In this version of *Open Letters*, Semmelweis presented a daunting review of the history of puerperal fever,
laying out the details of epidemics in more than forty European cities, spanning an era from 1600 to 1860. He then offered a tedious
recapitulation of his path to enlightenment and the development of
his doctrine.

Next he launched into an attack on two of his favorite targets—
Scanzoni and Carl Braun. He charged Scanzoni, along with the majority of European obstetricians, of sharing in the murder of gravid
women and their unborn, even though fifteen years had passed since
he had so clearly elucidated the cause of puerperal fever. Semmelweis charged both Scanzoni and Braun of quietly adopting his antiseptic safeguards at the very same time that they were preaching
against the doctrine to their obstetrical students. Both were just too
dishonest to admit it. Since Scanzoni had kept his students in the
dark, both as a teacher and writer, he, along with the majority of
professors, was an accomplice in the massacre perpetrated on gravid
women throughout Europe. This wholesale neglect of the *Lehre* was
"for me . . . an urgent summons to work vigorously for the propagation of the truth, in order to bring the atrocious waste of human life
to an end as soon as possible."[32]

As regards Braun, Semmelweis disparaged him for his soaring
mortality rates in Vienna and for the generally duplicitous manner
in which he argued his case. Braun could write against the doctrine
in one publication while sounding like a Semmelweis disciple in
another. In *Maternity Clinics*, Braun proclaimed that childbed fever,
or pyemia, was caused by the "inoculation of cadaver poison and
by transmission of septic exudates . . . it is the strictest duty of the
physician to see to it that the healthy puerperae are separated completely from the individuals ill with a zymotic disease . . . . and never to permit an examination or an operation on a pregnant, in labor
or puerperal woman when the medical attendant has, a short time
before, had dealings with parts of a cadaver or septic exudates."[33]

So, somewhere along the line in Braun's world, puerperal fever
had become an infectious disease, and precautions against cadavers
were warranted, after all. Extending his frustration with Braun to all
of the European professors of obstetrics, Semmelweis then divulged
his plan to take his case before the public:

I will, in order to save from Childbed Fever in the lying-in hospitals at least those women giving birth in this geographical
area, turn to the public . . . and I will say: father of the family,
do you know what it means to summon a [practitioner] . . . to
your wife, who needs assistance in her delivery? It is as if you

are putting your wife and your yet unborn child into mortal danger. And if you do not want to be a widower, and if you do not want your as yet unborn child to be inoculated with the germ of death, and in order that your child should not lose its mother, then buy with a few pennies some chlorinated lime, pour some water on it, and do not permit the [practitioners] . . . to carry out any internal examinations on your wife until the [practitioners] . . . have washed their hands in chlorine in your presence, and even then do not permit the [practitioners] . . . to examine internally until you yourself have become convinced by feeling their hands that the [practitioners] . . . have washed long enough so their hands have become slippery.[34]

Semmelweis cautioned potential fathers not to blame the individual practitioner who, out of ignorance, puts the expectant wife in danger: "The fault lies with the professors of obstetrics, from whom the [practitioners] . . . learned, and which professors did not teach the [practitioners] . . . to prevent the preventable absorption fever of the puerperal period of women, which is caused by preventable infections from without. I hope the public, which is in need of help, will be more educable than the professors of obstetrics."[35]

Before closing, Semmelweis had a score to settle with a biased disciple of Braun, Karl Patruban, prominent editor of an Austrian medical journal. Following an 1855 epidemic in Vienna, Braun had deceptively stated that chloride washings had been of no effect, after he had put them into use too late, well after the epidemic had peaked. Patruban wrote of Braun's "[h]ighly praiseworthy precautionary measures effected by the worthy director of the I clinic," and declared "what wicked deceptions Professor Semmelweis of Pest has indulged in relative to the infallibility of his prophylactic measures, and that it was absolutely untimely to disseminate those two notorious *Open Letters*, by whose contents the author has condemned himself."[36]

In fact, it was Braun who had deceived Patruban about the details of the preventive measures and his delay in instituting the chloride washings. Semmelweis responded that "The wicked deception in relation to the infallibility of my prophylactic measures is therefore not on my part, but rather on the part of Professor Patruban, and the fraud is on the part of Carl Braun."[37]

Semmelweis's *Open Letters to Professors* totaled ninety-two pages. It ended abruptly with the simple statement, "continuation and conclusion to follow."[38] But, it was never to be.

Public Reception

Not only were Semmelweis's contemporaries highly critical of him and his *Letters*, but he fared little better with his translators posthumously. Sounding like echoes of the critics of *Aetiology*, two Semmelweis scholars, Sherwin Nuland and Ferenc Gyorgyey, who were the first to translate all of Semmelweis's *Letters* from German into English, alluded to the difficulties posed by the author's "idiosyncratic personality" and his "reckless disregard for the usual conventions of literary style." They made no improvements or corrections to Semmelweis's literary style, translating it as accurately as possible.[39] The criticisms that translator Frank Murphy had previously leveled at *Aetiology*, that the author was "egotistic and bellicose," with an underlying paranoia, are evident, as well, in *Letters*. While Semmelweis's pain, bitterness, and sarcasm are readily apparent to the modern reader of English, *Letters* is perfectly lucid as the author makes point after cogent point.

The heavy-handed, impolitic reproaches that Semmelweis leveled at his enemies in *Letters* proved shocking not only to his opponents but to nearly all who read them. His intemperate, *ad hominem* attacks aimed at his critics, some even directed at the venerated Virchow, offended many of Semmelweis's own followers. Opponents, especially those who had been the targets of his criticism, called the letters hateful, clamorous, disorganized, contemptible, and . . . "extravagantly fanciful, the work of an obsessed maniac."[40] But such charges neither bothered nor surprised the author, who was only interested in getting his points across to as wide an audience as possible. Why would he care if he offended the feelings of those Philistines who had been so unfair to him?

Wilhelm Scanzoni and Carl Braun ignored Semmelweis's assaults in their entirety. Whether they familiarized themselves with his criticisms or not, neither uttered a word in defense of the charges leveled in either *Aetiology* or *Letters*. With all the criticism other physicians directed at Semmelweis's literary excesses, no need existed.

Semmelweis after Letters

As Semmelweis struggled with his depression and lack of acceptance by his colleagues, good news arrived on July 4, 1863, in the form of a letter from a Professor Hugenberger of St. Petersburg, Russia. Included were the proceedings of five meetings held by their medical society titled "The Etiology and Prophylaxis of Puerperal Fever." Hugenberger wrote, "You will see from this how many followers you have in the Far North, and how strongly the younger men support you." As the society's discussions progressed, it became apparent that Semmelweis enjoyed their strongest support, except for a few who still adhered to Kiwisch's epidemic miasmatic theory. At the meetings' conclusion, the society wisely passed a resolution requiring all obstetrical caregivers to utilize the chloride regimen.

Semmelweis was visibly pleased with such positive news. For a time he appeared generally soothed, his mood less angry. He happily contributed several articles regarding the St. Petersburg affair to the *Medical Weekly*. But with those essays, his writing efforts on the entire subject of puerperal fever were forever concluded. It had become all too evident that Semmelweis appeared pained when colleagues sought from him a better explanation of some nuanced or controversial point in his doctrine. Answering the same points over and over again had become mentally debilitating. Between his exhausted state and his angst provoked by *Aetiology* and *Open Letters*, he had lost all his will to expound further on the subject. What more could he say? He finally handed the task of defending the finer points of his theory over to Marko. To Marie and those in Semmelweis's inner circle, the image he projected of a physically and mentally spent man was troubling.

Semmelweis may have been through proselytizing and defending his theory, but his mind remained generally clear. While limiting his efforts to less contentious subjects, such as gynecology, he continued on with his writing. He was in the process of writing a textbook on gynecology, a task that he would never finish. He was competent enough to publish what would be his last article, "The Operative Treatment of the Ovarian Cyst," in the *Medical Weekly* on July 18, 1865.[41] Despite his mental exhaustion, Semmelweis remained active in university affairs, including time-consuming seats on multiple committees. In the early 1860s, he directed the university's smallpox vaccination program. He was not only responsible for quality control and disbursement of the vaccine to physicians, but also for delivering weekly lectures espousing the desirability of vaccination and immunity. One activity that proved both physically and emotionally draining to him was his assignment as economic superintendant of the medical faculty. In that capacity, he ran the university hospital laundry, nearly a full time job in itself. As director, he had to pay strict attention to detail, much as if he were the managing owner of the enterprise. Not only was he personally accountable for any financial shortages that might arise, he was also responsible for meeting payroll, quality control, employee relations, delivery of bed linens, and so on. In a facility that not infrequently neglected paying its employees, Semmelweis would, on occasion, pay them out of his own pocket so that they might put food on their tables. With his insistence on clean bed linens for all hospital patients, it was sometimes difficult to do business with the lowest bidder while maintaining high quality control. As a consequence, he was often censured for his "extravagant" operating budget. Semmelweis begged university authorities to be relieved of this duty, only to be consistently rebuffed.[42]

Even after publication of *Aetiology* and *Letters*, other mental strains continued, exacerbated, if not caused in part, by his onerous workload and the highly contentious atmosphere that typified faculty meetings. Of course, Semmelweis's own bellicose attitude did nothing to diminish those tensions. Ideological conflicts within the Pest faculty, centering mainly upon medievalism versus modernism in medicine, provided plenty of rhetorical fodder, reminiscent of the Old versus New School tensions in Vienna a decade earlier. Even though Lajos Tognio, Pest's professor of pathology and pharmacology, had died in 1848, his moral authority favoring medical medievalism still held sway with the old, conservative wing of the faculty. Tognio could not bear the thought of introducing more enlightened reforms into the university, especially in the area of medical research. Janos Balassa, who headed Pest's more modern faction, had to contend with Tognio's continuing influence. Semmelweis, typically in the thick of the resultant debates, could become instantly enraged when confronted in argumentation, especially if he considered his adversaries to be professionally slovenly, dishonest, or disloyal. Faculty members, repulsed by his anger and his refusal to consider an opposing point of view, began avoiding him out of a combination of dislike and fear.[43]

The most distinctly identifiable change in Semmelweis's spirit occurred between 1862 and 1863. Duka pointed to one of the critical precipitating elements of the man's angst: "Semmelweis felt that he had grasped a great truth which had been gradually evolved out of a long series of observations and much concentrated thought."[44] But now it was all falling apart. Even as he engaged in one of his favorite pursuits, lecturing to his medical students, it became painfully evident that he was navigating too near the margins of mental normality. He had become so obsessed with the topic of puerperal infection that he could hardly keep from refracting every subject in medicine, every mental challenge, through the lens of his *Lehre*. If addressing a subject unrelated to puerperal fever, such as ovarian tumors, Semmelweis somehow managed to swing the topic over to an exposition of his *Lehre*, hoping to make converts of his students. As he became increasingly emotional laying out the facts supporting his theory, empathetic students watched in anxious sadness as their respected professor brushed up all too close to his mental breaking point.[45]

Other manifestations of Semmelweis's chronic depression were evident. Though he had become aware that other prominent obstetricians, such as Joseph Spaeth, had finally converted to his theory—with the single exception of Hugenberger—it seemed to give him little pleasure. Concerned associates, such as Marko, Hirschler, and Arneth, all agreed. They had never seen their friend so moody, so apathetic, so mentally exhausted—a sinister omen of things to come.

Illness and Descent

With the completion of *Aetiology* and all his *Open Letters*, Semmelweis's more immediate stresses may have been diminished, but he still chafed from other strains. His general zest for polemics, an activity that he never relished, was definitely on the wane—another manifestation of his mental fatigue. When anyone voiced disagreement regarding his doctrine, he could still muster the energy to become livid, but his rage was less sustained. Apathy coupled with an increased sense of persecution became more clearly evident. Semmelweis did continue with other less stressful activities. He was busy working on a textbook of obstetrics, as well as his handbook of gynecology. He directed more energy into his gynecologic practice and university matters, lecturing to medical societies while remaining active in their functions. And, he had made some progress within his own workplace. After enduring his struggles with a doubting and hostile hospital staff, he had, by 1860, finally converted them to his side. His mortality rate for 1859–1860 was an admirable 0.9 percent. The staff, after viewing firsthand the direct effects of his enlightened diligence, could no longer dismiss his methods as impractical or too cumbersome.

Despite that single improvement in his workplace environment, Semmelweis's moods continued to be ever more autonomous as his manic periods became increasingly bizarre.[1] Writer Alfred Hegar, obstetrics professor at Freiburg, described pathetic street scenes in which Semmelweis, confronted complete strangers, laymen with no medical knowledge whatsoever, argued passionately for his doctrine as the puzzled strangers timidly backed away, scratching their heads. On at least one occasion, he conducted a soapbox oration on his doctrine in a park setting, provoking sarcastic epithets from passersby. Other equally disturbing behaviors emerged, such as his use of loud and obscene language and excessive use of alcohol, both completely out of character for this normally gentle man. At other times he displayed "childish" behavior that was disturbing to both his patients and colleagues.[2] During his normal, happier years, Semmelweis had always displayed an indifference to monetary concerns, feeling a continuing obligation to serve the public over himself. His assets were so marginal when he did die that his family was left nearly destitute. Yet, as he waxed manic during his working years, his persona commonly turned expansive as he began boasting of his vast wealth and extensive possessions, a signature trait of the manic phase of bipolar illness.

Hypersexual activity surfaced as another manifestation of his mania. Immediately after making love with Maria, Semmelweis, obviously unsatiated, would indulge in autoeroticism.[3] Other forms of sexual excess became evident later. As obstetrician and writer Sillo-Seidl conducted his research in the 1970s, he discovered that an archivist, Professor Jantsch, at the Institute of Medical History in Vienna, had become aware of some sexual indiscretions on Semmelweis's part that were, reportedly, so scandalous that Jantsch considered them to be unmentionable. According to Sillo-Seidl, Jantsch made any full, unfettered access to Semmelweis's records impossible, in an effort to avoid further damage to the man's reputation. Though no specific details of time and place were offered, records indicated that, during some of Semmelweis's manic episodes, he had purportedly groped women and at other times indulged in onanism. Jantsch, until finally confronted by Sillo-Seidl, had kept this "objectional [sic] material" from full public view, feeling that it would "not [be] desirable for the public to find out that Semmelweis had groped women under their skirts."[4] Setting the feelings of the victims aside, such behavior would have, indeed, been an unspeakably shocking and ironic violation of public trust for this obstetrician who, as some type of undiagnosed eccentric, would still have been considered responsible for his own actions. But, when viewed more appropriately in the modern context of an honorable man suffering through the throes of an acute manic phase of a chronic bipolar condition, it is more readily understood—a sad event over which he had no control.

As Semmelweis's manic episodes eventually resolved, desolation and darkness followed—the depths of depression. Since depressive episodes are less flamboyant than manias, biographers have been able to elicit even less concerning the details in Semmelweis's case. Clinical depression, the type endured by manic-depressive patients, is far worse than situational depression, a condition from which all people suffer on occasion, whether occasioned by romantic, financial, or other setbacks. Sufferers of true clinical depression, with its constant, painful tedium, invariably claim that the condition defies description. One has to live through such an episode to fully appreciate its horrors. All words, comparisons, even metaphors fail to adequately convey the feelings endured. Dread and desperation are often so intense that sufferers feel compelled to commit sudden irrational acts, such as jumping off rooftops or hurling themselves under the wheels of an oncoming train. According to psychiatrist Kay Redfield Jamison, herself a sufferer, life is "flat, hollow, and unendurable . . . awful beyond words or sounds or images."[5]

Remarkably, despite suffering from such episodes, Semmelweis continued to work over the years, through every permutation of his troubled moods. In fact, according to psychiatrist Hagop Akiskal, such behavior typifies the person with a depressive temperament. Psychiatric authorities describe such depressives as "hard working, dependable, sensitive to the suffering and needs of others . . . suitable for jobs that require long periods of devotion to meticulous detail." Such individuals commonly shoulder all the burdens of their jobs without experiencing its pleasures.[6] Semmelweis, conducting his revolutionary research, stealing hours at his desk writing *Aetiology* and *Letters* while pursuing his onerous workload, fits the template well.

Semmelweis's more precipitous decline began on a fateful Thursday evening, July 13, 1865, when he and his family attended a dinner party in a suburb of Budapest. Although details are sparse, Semmelweis reportedly "behaved in such an extraordinary manner during a meal, and shewed such an unnatural and remarkable facial expression" that it not only caused a premature break-up of the party, but it left Maria greatly alarmed.[7] While she had become accustomed to simply ignoring his unending eccentricities over the past several years, it suddenly dawned on her, as they headed for home, that her husband was going insane. Later, when she related the episode to Marko, he was hardly surprised. Marko had long recognized the great amount of stress that Semmelweis's work on puerperal fever was placing upon him. On more than one occasion, he had pleaded with his old friend to forget about puerperal fever—for his own good. But that was akin to asking Mozart to give up composing because it made him drink excessively. Semmelweis's identity was so tied up with his *Lehre* that giving it up was completely out of the question.

Then, in late July, approximately a week after the troubling dinner scene, Semmelweis suffered an acute mental breakdown that rendered him incompetent. Details are fragmentary, but it is known that three of Budapest's finest physicians, under the direction of Janos Balassa, were summoned to Semmelweis's aid. One explanation of the man's acute descent, attributed to old friend and former Semmelweis student Josef Fleischer, arose several years after Semmelweis's death. Although the tale has never been fully corroborated, it has gained a certain level of credence, and by this late date, it remains the only explanation in existence. According to Fleischer, Semmelweis attended a gathering of the Committee of Professors on July 21, a fateful meeting in which he had been assigned two tasks. First, he was expected to deliver a short address concerning the appointment of a faculty member to a new position.[8] Secondly, he planned to petition the committee for an increase in his own salary. Records indicate that Semmelweis did, in fact, receive his salary increase a few weeks after the meeting, casting some doubt on Fleischer's following account. According to Fleischer, when Semmelweis's time to speak arrived, he rose from his seat, walked silently up to the podium, and slowly pulled a sheet of paper from his pants pocket. Without looking up he began reading—but his remarks had nothing to do with his assigned subject. He was, instead, reading from the text of the Midwives' Oath, their solemn pledge of professional conduct.[9] Puzzled by the inappropriate comments, faculty members began exchanging uneasy glances, while allowing him some additional time. Perhaps he was making a point via some circuitous route. But soon it was undeniable—Semmelweis was completely irrational. Professor Balassa took charge, walking up to the podium and, along with several other members, gently helped Semmelweis to the nearest seat. The most celebrated, albeit controversial, member of the Pest faculty had made his final official statement—and it was pitifully nonsensical. Balassa invited the aforementioned physicians, Janos Wagner and Janos Bokai, to join Semmelweis's treatment team. Why would Balassa, instead of perhaps Marko, Semmelweis's closest ally, take charge? Even though Balassa and Semmelweis were colleagues in Pest, Balassa, a surgeon, had never fully accepted Semmelweis's *Lehre*. Although the two were mutually collegial, they were not on the most intimate of terms.[10]

After accompanying Semmelweis home, Balassa's team sedated and phlebotomized their patient. Some of his early behavior, such as walking around the house completely undressed, was disturbing enough that two physicians were assigned to monitor him continuously. Despite his mounting problems, Semmelweis still loved to play with his children, especially the youngest, Antoinette. As he swung her about, nervous eyes monitored his every move.[11] Balassa anxiously observed his patient over a period of several days, watching Semmelweis's sensorium as it cycled between confusion and lucidity. It took him but a few days to become confident that his patient was getting progressively worse. During one moment of clarity, Semmelweis admitted to Maria that he knew something inside his head was not right. He needed help. With the aid of Balassa's group, the couple came to a decision. Semmelweis would first undergo a more thorough medical evaluation in Budapest and then travel to the Spa at Grafenberg, in southern Germany. Not only were their baths therapeutic, but the cold water treatment program they offered was very popular, as well. If nothing else, a prolonged rest at the spa, away from the vexations of daily life, should be beneficial in itself.

It is curious that Janos Bokai, rather than Balassa or Wagner, would be the only physician selected to perform that first thorough medical evaluation. Balassa could have just as easily gone outside the group and selected from a broad array of readily available medical experts in Budapest.[12] Bokai was Semmelweis's old pediatrician friend, and head of Hungary's largest children's hospital. He would hardly seem the first choice to assess an adult problem. After first performing a general examination, Bokai declared all to be normal.

Yet, in 1906, in an interview granted forty years after the fact, Maria related how Semmelweis, in early July 1865, had cut his right middle finger during some sort of obstetrical operation. He spent the ensuing days treating the wound but with little success. By making no specific mention of Semmelweis's extremities, fingers in particular, Bokai was innocently adding to a mystery that would later raise its head.

Next came Bokai's mental evaluation. For this information, he relied heavily on those closest to Semmelweis, including Maria and her family. Bokai duly noted that Maria's side of the family commonly referred to Semmelweis as "the crazy Naczi."[13] He made note of Semmelweis's longstanding social problems, such as his generally bellicose attitude, his difficulty with anger control, and his inability to tolerate contradictory opinions. Semmelweis had, as well, recently been concerned, to the point of obsession, with the notion of translating *Aetiology* into Hungarian in hopes of gaining acceptance into the Hungarian Academy.[14] Bokai also uncovered something new: his patient had been suffering from narcolepsy over the past several years. Accenting Semmelweis's recent confusional episodes, Bokai concluded that his patient suffered from an acute mental disturbance that has "brought us to distance our unfortunate colleague from his present surroundings and to transfer him to such conditions that, under the medical direction of a specialist, might work favorably on his mental disturbance."[15] In effect, he was declaring Semmelweis insane. According to German obstetrician Georg Sillo-Seidl, Bokai concluded his exam by compiling a list of signs and symptoms, in summarized form, providing a "textbook picture" of a mental condition synonymous with manic-depressive psychosis, without specifically using that term.[16] Bokai's failure to use the term gives further evidence that manic-depressive illness was not yet generally appreciated. Even after Bokai's declaration, the trio of physicians continued to administer to Semmelweis in his home, over the next week, but with little effect. With Semmelweis's confusion and passionate outbreaks worsening, the trio became increasingly convinced that caring for him in a home setting was impossible.

It was at this time that his treatment plan took a different path, a peculiar turn leading some biographers to raise the possibility of a conspiracy. When Sillo-Seidl wrote his 1978 biography, he was especially intent on uncovering the obviously large gaps of information concerning the last days of Semmelweis—in particular those details surrounding his 1865 illness and hospitalization. These records, inexplicably unavailable to previous researchers, lend further credence to prior suspicions of a conspiracy against Semmelweis. Even today, despite the efforts of scholars like Sillo-Seidl and others, details of Semmelweis's illness and death remain clouded in suspicion. Why would such public records, some even secured under lock and key, not be readily available? Sillo-Seidl pursued them through the Vienna Archives.[17] And, for those information-seeking readers of English, noted Semmelweis authority Dr. K. Codell Carter, provided new material in 1995 by translating most of the work surrounding Semmelweis's confinement and final days. The following information, from these two sources, helps explain Semmelweis's peculiar fate.

Sillo-Seidl asserts that Semmelweis's colleagues considered his overall behavior, of late, to have become intolerably peculiar and embarrassing. They wanted him gone, removed from the scene, even though it was arguable whether or not they had sufficient evidence that he was, in fact, mentally deranged.[18] Suddenly confronted with Semmelweis's purportedly acute mental deterioration, the three involved physicians had been granted a gift. They sensed a unique opportunity—a perfect time for getting rid of their bellicose colleague in a manner that would have all the appearances of legitimacy. Institutionalization was the answer.[19]

On July 29, 1865, Janos Balassa composed a letter committing Semmelweis to a Viennese mental institution: "The undersigned confirm herewith that Professor Dr. Ignaz Semmelweis of the R[oyal] University at Pest has been burdened for three weeks by an ongoing disturbance of his mental state which implies on the one hand removal from his usual surroundings and from the practice of his vocation and on the other hand suitable supervision and medical care; which can be achieved most surely in an institution for the mentally ill; therefore the undersigned recommend his accommodation in the I[mperial]. R[oyal]. State Mental Institution. Pest 29 July 1865."[20] All three men, Wagner, Balassa, and Bokai, in that order, signed the formal letter certifying Semmelweis as mentally incompetent. Despite the reference to a Viennese mental asylum, the trio had believed, initially, that Semmelweis would be best cared for in a nearby modern psychiatric facility, the Schwartzer Institute of Buda. If Semmelweis's deteriorating mental state was as urgent as they claimed, then seeking treatment locally would have seemed the most prudent course. But, as Sillo-Seidl contended, they soon discovered a problem. Schwartzer and Semmelweis knew each other. They had not only been fellow students in Vienna, but their friendship went all the way back to their youth. Sillo-Seidl believed that, in all likelihood, Schwartzer would have neither diagnosed mental illness in his old friend, nor have considered admission to his facility to be appropriate. That brought up the option of choosing an institution in Vienna instead. Yet that posed its own set of problems. If Semmelweis's mental state were truly deteriorating, could he even make the longer trip by rail? One other major problem: Semmelweis might be suffering from some as yet undiagnosed illness, but his mind, contrary to Bokai's contention, was, save for some episodic confusion, generally intact. How could he be convinced to willingly enter a mental institution?[21]

Keeping Semmelweis himself completely in the dark, the group hatched an alternative plan sometime between July 28 and 29. This scheme depended entirely on the cooperation of several individuals, both in Budapest and Vienna, whom Semmelweis trusted.[22] Two of the three obvious trusted intimates of Semmelweis were Maria, and in Vienna, Ferdinand Hebra. Whether or not Sillo-Seidl's assertions are true, both Maria and Hebra must have possessed foreknowledge of the upcoming events. However, in Maria's defense, she had been led to believe that her husband would be admitted to a private Viennese mental facility run by two individuals: chief physician and Semmelweis's former fellow student Dr. Riedel; and the asylum's director, Dr. Mildner. Semmelweis only understood that he and his party, as planned earlier, would be traveling by train to Grafenburg for treatment. He and Maria, however, would make one brief stop en route, in Vienna, for a visit with his trusted old friend, Hebra. Somehow Hebra had been notified of the plans by wire, but exactly what information had been shared with him is unknown.[23] On July 29, the same day Semmelweis had been certified as mentally incompetent, his party boarded the Saturday night train in Budapest for the overnight trip to Vienna. On board were Semmelweis; Maria with

Antoinette, their unweaned one-year-old child; Maria's uncle; and Istvan Bathory, Semmelweis's assistant in Budapest.

Sillo-Seidl charges that Bathory was likely another "trusted" third party involved in the conspiracy. He had just completed his two-year assistantship under Semmelweis in Pest, but Semmelweis had not reappointed him for the usual second term. In fact, his successor was already in place. Whether or not Bathory harbored any animus towards Semmelweis is unknown. Yet, why would travel plans include someone who had no discernible reason to accompany the family on such a sensitive and personal mission?

As the party arrived at Vienna's station on Sunday morning, there was Hebra on the platform extending a warm welcome to them all. The party split into two separate cabs for the trip to Hebra's home nearby, where all were received by Hebra's wife, Johanna. Upon recognizing Johanna, Semmelweis greeted her warmly saying, "Here I am again, an ill lad! But Ferdinand will make me well again. He is the only one whom I trust."[24] As the party intermingled, getting re-acquainted, Hebra drew Semmelweis aside from the group, suggesting that now would be a propitious time for the two of them to tour his new, private sanitarium. Hebra then made an offer. If Semmelweis were so inclined, he could even be accommodated there in his own private cold water-cure facility.[25] Semmelweis readily agreed to the proposal from his trusted old friend. As he climbed back into the cab, he asked Maria, "Aren't you coming?"

"She and the girl will stay with me," answered Johanna.

Suddenly recalling how he had attended Johanna's delivery back in 1847, Semmelweis shouted back at his former patient, "Do you still remember how I called to you: It is a boy!?" After exchanging farewells, the cab door closed, and off he went sitting in between Hebra and Bathory, looking forward to the visit.[26] But Hebra's supposed private sanitarium was nothing more than the Lower Austrian Mental Home, a large public insane asylum on Lazarethgasse, near Vienna's General Hospital.

Far from being an enlightened institution functioning along the lines of French reformer Pinel, this facility still languished in hopeless medievalism. It warehoused nearly seven hundred inmates with maladies ranging from the mentally ill to those who were nothing

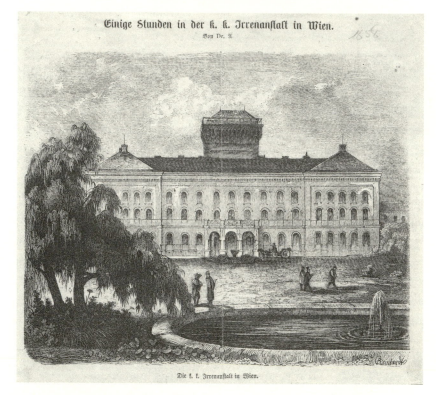

Einige Stunden in der k. k. Irrenanstalt in Wien.
Von Dr. A.

Die k. k. Irrenanstalt in Wien.

Figure 22. Vienna's Lower Austrian Mental Asylum in 1858, a large, unenlightened public institution designed to warehouse any and all intractable social problems. An etching by Carl August Reinhardt. Courtesy of Vienna University's Josephinum.

more than a burden to their families, money scammers, gamblers, bank draft forgers—in short, anyone with a significant social or mental problem.[27] Yet, Semmelweis entered the facility with his "trusted old friend," blissfully unaware of what he was about to encounter.

Why such a facility, certainly not one of the empire's finest, was chosen for someone of Semmelweis's prominence remains a mystery, unless Sillo-Seidl's conspiratorial charges are correct. As they arrived at the asylum, Bathory, playing the role of caregiver, reached into his bag and presented to institutional authorities the certificate of insanity signed by the three men. Bathory, his role apparently completed, then disappeared from the scene. Sillo-Seidl pointed to yet another curious fact. Although Semmelweis had recently terminated Bathory from his assistantship, the Pest faculty had just awarded him with a two-year trip abroad, an assignment he would begin immediately upon his return to Budapest.[28]

The three—Hebra, the uncle, and Semmelweis—began their tour, ambling from one ward to the next, accompanied by multiple staff members. Semmelweis reportedly showed great interest in the facility, engaging staff members in spirited conversation as they moved about. As they entered one particular unoccupied single room, Semmelweis's eyes were drawn immediately to the heavy metal bars on the windows. Puzzled, he inquired as to their necessity. They are for "safety's sake," replied an aide.[29] As a member of the asylum staff deliberately engaged him in conversation inside the room, Semmelweis appeared to accept that explanation. Sensing his distracted state, Hebra and the uncle slowly moved towards the door, hoping to slip out unnoticed. But Semmelweis, seeing the two out of the corner of his eye, sensed that some danger was afoot. He made a quick move towards the door to join them, only to be surrounded and restrained by the guards. Realizing that he had been duped, Semmelweis reacted true to his mercurial temperament, screaming accusations and flailing wildly. Naturally, the greater his resistance, the more certain were the guards of his insanity. Finally, six attendants were able to secure Semmelweis in a straitjacket—the operation completed. Fully restrained and locked in his room, he was imprisoned, completely neutralized in a darkened cell reserved for "maniacs."[30]

Lower Austrian Mental Asylum

Aside from Semmelweis remaining in restraints for most of Sunday, no other information is available regarding his first day of admission. The next day, Monday, Chief Physician Riedel returned from his vacation. When attendants informed him of Semmelweis's admission, he hurried to his former friend's bedside, anxious to better understand the circumstances leading to his admission. Semmelweis, whether confused or still seething from his prior restraints, greeted the chief physician with a brisk slap across his face. Enraged, Riedel had Semmelweis placed back into his straitjacket and tied to the bed, where he reportedly remained for several days.[1] Exactly what transpired the rest of that Monday, like Sunday, remains unclear.

In fact, most subsequent events involving Semmelweis's stay at the asylum remain nebulous due to poor documentation. Hospital chart entries, recovered years later by Sillo-Seidl, had been organized serially from the day of entry onward. But, strangely, charted entries exist for only nine of Semmelweis's total fifteen days of confinement. Other notations, crossed out with corrections entered over them, are of dubious credibility. Whether such ambiguities were purposeful or merely a result of sloppy record keeping at the time of his hospital stay is not entirely clear. The records retrieved, however, were complete enough to clarify the fate that awaited Semmelweis. Further examination of these records proved instructive, raising additional questions both as to their accuracy and reliability. Instead of making journal entries on an ongoing daily basis, handwriting analysis indicates that all entries, from July 31 to August 12, were most likely written after the fact, all at one sitting, by the same hand, with the same writing instrument.[2] Additionally, Sillo-Seidl expected to find the names of Mildner and Riedel all over the chart, since they were the two rendering care to this famous patient. Instead, only three incidental references were made using the impersonal, generic term "doctors' visit," but the names of Mildner or Riedel never appear inside the chart.[3] Did these two men, whether for legal, ethical, or other reasons, not want their names associated in any way with this dubious case?

On Monday, the same day as Riedel's memorable visit to Semmelweis, Maria, accompanied by her uncle, came to the asylum most anxious for an update on her husband's condition. Aides informed her that he had fallen "into a fit of delirium so that six attendants could scarcely hold him back."[4] She did have a meeting with Riedel, who gently informed her that any thoughts of a visit with Ignaz would, at the present time, be absolutely impossible. In her distraught state, with a nursing child on her arm and an apparent wall thrown up between her and her husband, she felt powerless. Frustrated, she returned to Budapest with the rest of the party the next day, where she reportedly remained bedridden for the next six weeks. Sadly, Maria would never see her husband again. There is no evidence that any family member ever visited Semmelweis, or even inquired as to his condition, during his entire stay in the asylum. Considering that Maria's side of the family had referred to him with the denigrating term "crazy Naczi," their apparent lack of concern hardly seems surprising.

The first actual entry, illegibly dated either July 30 or 31, 1865, but soon after admission, described the patient as "spirited, but not illogical." He reportedly spoke continuously, mostly about his field of obstetrics. He was presumably febrile with a "hot head," and a pulse of 120. Aides noted a dark bluish-red spot, covered by reactive skin, on the radial (outer) edge of the last phalanx of the right middle finger. It could have been a contusion or the early stages of gangrene. When aides questioned Semmelweis as to its origin, he stated that it had developed spontaneously. He had neither cut nor infected himself during any operation that he could recall. Entries before August 3 duly noted that the wound had spread into the adjacent knuckle joint.[5] A day or two after admission, when attendants finally released Semmelweis from the straight jacket that had been placed on admission, they noticed dark spots on his right forearm that appeared to be gangrenous.[6] Except for applying a dressing to his finger, aides rendered no treatment of any sort to either his hand or forearm.

After attendants observed Semmelweis for hours and were convinced that he was less combative, they removed his restraints, whereupon he took off all his clothes and lay on the floor as though attempting to get rid of bodily heat. He next laid in the bed with a wash basin given to him for bathing, but he spilled it in his bed on three separate occasions. Later he appeared delirious, again speaking continuously about obstetrical topics, referring repeatedly to the Hungarian Academy and his intent to translate Siebold's work. Other early entries indicated some level of confusion when he stated, "I was in the Kartner-Gate Theater, Tomorrow I will travel to Grafenberg."[7] Over the ensuing days, he remained confused and restive much of the time, with incessant aimless activity. During one such early episode he made a vigorous attempt to jump out the window. Aides reacted by consigning him once again to his straitjacket where he remained for the majority of his confinement.

Hospital staff did not bother to make any entries for August 3.

By August 4, five days after admission, Semmelweis appeared weak and generally tremulous. He often lay supine, gnashing his teeth while continuouusly throwing himself about, rolling side to side.[8] When aides refused his request to walk in the corridor he became so agitated that three attendants could barely control him. Attendants then noted a new development: "asthmatic breathing." He was experiencing air hunger, with heavy panting and marked shortness of breath. Not only had the lesion on his finger become clearly "gangrenous," but multiple boils (furuncles) with gas gangrene were now evident on his thighs, as well.[9] Asylum personnel merely continued with their passive observations, never rendering treatment of any sort.

Incredibly, on August 5, Joseph Skoda, the same Skoda who had crossed off his former student as an "ingrate," paid him a visit. Semmelweis was reportedly lucid enough to recognize his old professor, carry on a conversation, and even convey to Skoda his desire to become a member of the Hungarian Academy.[10] Surely Skoda, arguably the best diagnostician in all of Europe, had to have recognized what was going on with Semmelweis, if not politically, at least medically. As unlikely as was Skoda's visit, why did other so called friends avoid visiting Semmelweis? Where were the likes of Hebra, Balassa, Bokai, Wagner, and even Markusovsky?

By August 7, Semmelweis's sensorium was reported as nonsensical, "frenzied and combative." His middle finger was even more gangrenous. He had boils "everywhere on the extremities." His breathing had not only become more labored, but aides noted, as well, that he had multiple episodes of turning dusky-blue.

On August 12, Semmelweis was reported as being obstinate to all. By afternoon he recognized no one and "speaks stammering nonsense."

Hospital notes of August 13 described Semmelweis as having a persisting tachycardia and nearly continual breathing difficulties. He remained generally immobile, incommunicative, with vacuous, glassy eyes, half open. His lower jaw reportedly hung down, mouth agape, revealing a tongue "hard as a board."[11] Now, two weeks post-admission, a large abscess was evident on the left side of his chest. The observer surmised that pyemia must be present. That same evening, Semmelweis died quietly in his cell with no further physical developments being recorded.

Even in those terminal few days, when it was obvious that Semmelweis was close to death, there is no evidence that his caregivers ever rendered any sort of treatment, either of a comforting or therapeutic nature. Despite the attending staff's knowledge of Semmelweis's Roman Catholic faith, no priest ever made a bedside visit. Even when death was imminent, he received no last rites of the church.[12] This pioneering medical scientist was, in essence, warehoused with asylum personnel casually observing physical changes along the way, as life slowly ebbed from his body.

Authorities wasted little time in proceeding with post-death necessities. On the very next day, August 14, Semmelweis's body was removed to the Pathologic Institute, the same old facility in which he had performed hundreds, if not thousands, of autopsies. Now he, like Kolletschka eight years before, would be subjected to the same ritual. One of Rokitansky's assistants, Gustav Scheutauer, performed the post-mortem exam. The most dramatic findings did not even require an incision: linear pressure injuries corresponding to the strap marks of his straitjacket were evident on his arms and trunk. Multiple boils covered his body. The large "fist sized" abscess occupying the muscles of his left chest exuded "stinking gases." It penetrated deeply, through the chest wall, resulting in a collapsed lung and a pus-filled chest cavity.

In addition, Scheutauer found changes of osteomyelitis (abscesses, in effect, with bacteria sequestered inside the bone) in Semmelweis's right elbow (olecranon) and middle finger. Examination of the left kidney revealed a "walnut sized" abscess.[13]

Semmelweis's nervous system revealed widespread hyperemia of the meninges (a vascular engorgement of the outer membranes covering his brain) and nonspecific changes consistent with acute inflammation. Frontal atrophy (wasting) was evident to the naked eye. Scheutauer's knife slices through the cerebral hemispheres revealed enlarged ventricles (the natural cavities holding cerebrospinal fluid). When viewed microscopically, the brain tissue proper revealed changes consistent with nonspecific inflammation. Scheutauer found only edema in the spinal cord (an abnormal amount of water residing within its tissues, rather than within the blood vessels).

Some Semmelweis scholars, such as Hegar and Benedek, believed that Semmelweis's injuries could only be explained as a result of beatings at the hands of hospital attendants. Benedek cites the findings of osteomyelitis in Semmelweis's second, third, and fourth metacarpal bones of his right hand, along with findings of generalized inflammation and scattered abscesses. He then declared, "It is obvious that these horrifying injuries were . . . the consequence of brutal beatings, tying down, trampling underfoot."[14] Writer Irvine Loudon, as well, alleged that it was "forcible restraint by the asylum attendants. Semmelweis was, in effect, bludgeoned to death and that 'brain disease' was a euphemism for brain injury."[15] In fact, the most striking autopsy findings were the generalized inflammatory infiltrates throughout his body, including the brain and spinal cord. Such findings are not consistent with traumatic origins, but rather with widespread infection—pyemia—the formal cause of Semmelweis's death. It is highly likely that Semmelweis did have some trauma inflicted on him as a consequence of forcible restraining, if not from gratuitous beatings. Such treatment was sadly all too common in mental institutions of that era.

With Semmelweis's numerous metastatic abscesses, it was evident that he was the victim of pyemia, a process that had begun slowly, but over a period of weeks transitioned from low virulence to fulminating, eventuating in his death. The question arises as to how long he might have suffered with some level of pyemia. Was the final infectious scenario all the result of his infected finger, which occurred some four to six weeks earlier? Or did it develop, as some claim, coincident with his asylum confinement? Finally, was he the victim of some other disease, especially general paralysis of the insane (neurosyphilis) as the formal pathologic diagnosis, newspaper obituaries, and some biographers claimed? Some adversaries of Semmelweis were only too eager to attribute his demise to neurosyphilis with its implication of some level of moral turpitude. In fact, syphilis was a significant occupational hazard for physicians, especially obstetricians. Not only did they deal with prostitutes and syphilitic patients on a near-daily basis, but they also performed internal examinations with their bare hands, decades before the advent of rubber gloves.

Hospital authorities again demonstrated great efficiency, wasting little time with the next step. Semmelweis was laid to rest on August 15 in Vienna's Schmelzer Cemetery, the former burial grounds of fighters who died in the Revolution of 1848. The burial was held early, only forty-eight hours after his death, and it was August, the month in which Europe shuts down for vacation. Friends may not have had sufficient time to attend his services. Still, when one considers Semmelweis's celebrated, albeit troubled, status, surprisingly few attended the service. Among those present from Vienna were Karl Rokitansky; recent convert Joseph Spaeth; and the Braun brothers, Carl and Gustav. No mention was made of either Skoda or Hebra being present.[16] From Budapest, only one person, Semmelweis's longtime friend Lajos Markusovsky, attended. No other colleague from the University of Pest paid their respects.

The medical press proved little more considerate than the medical community. His death was effectively ignored, save for a few brief announcements. Sadly, not one immediate or extended member of the Semmelweis family paid their respects at the service.[17] Maria later alleged that she became so ill after her husband's flamboyant deterioration that she had been confined to bed for six weeks. How-

ever, she later changed the family name, Semmelweis, to its Mag-
yarized form, "Szemerenyi." Was she embarrassed by the name, by
all of the sensation surrounding the perceived abrupt mental decline
of her husband, by the notoriety occasioned by her husband dying in
a lunatic asylum? When colleagues in Budapest, painfully familiar
of Semmelweis's eccentricities, heard that he had died in a mental institution, they found it not at all surprising. It fit the pattern.
Whether or not it was true or fair, he was perceived publicly as having died from a fulminating insanity.

Semmelweis had been a longtime member of two different prestigious Hungarian professional organizations. The first, the Hungarian Association of Physicians and Natural Scientists, led by Balassa, had a policy of delivering a commemorative address, within
the year, in recognition of any member who had died. Semmelweis
never received such an accolade. Similarly, rules of the Pest Association of Physicians mandated that a eulogy be delivered honoring any
member who had died within the past year. Semmelweis finally did
receive that recognition in the form of two short, formulaic sentenc-
es, although it came seven long years after his death.[18]

Marko, in his *Medical Weekly*, bid an unabashed, poignant good-
bye to his friend of more than two decades: "How unscrutable [*sic*]
the ways of providence are that a man who devoted his untiring efforts to studying a disease and succeeded in saving millions of lives
should have been visited by another shape of the same disease to
cut short his life and extinguish his energy. . . . It would be unfair
not to speak of his upright, honest stature, of his feeling heart, and
his goodwill to all men, although his manners may not always have
been smooth and balanced. . . . Professor Semmelweis was an upright, natural man, and it was impossible for him to be anything
else. Egotism and cringing were equally foreign to his noble soul: he
was a loyal friend and colleague."[19]

Whether the medical community at large just did not care about
Semmelweis, or was only too eager to relegate him to the past, remains a mystery. After 1865, whenever meetings on puerperal fever
were convened, the essence of Semmelweis's *Lehre* was usually presented as gospel, but always in a generic form, giving no recognition
to its author. Shortly after Semmelweis's death, two of his own University of Pest assistants applied for his professorial chair. But the

powerful Balassa, still agnostic regarding Semmelweis's *Lehre*, recommended Janos Diescher for the position, a man with absolutely no obstetrical training. As Diescher assumed his position, mortality rates rose six-fold over those of Semmelweis's usual 1 percent. At St. Rochus, the identical scenario played out with another Semmelweis replacement. As Waldheim noted, "Pest offered the sad spectacle of dividing his [Semmelweis's] responsibilities between two of his opponents who were outstanding only in respect to their insignificance."[20] In fact, Diescher's mortality rates remained so high that hospital authorities ultimately replaced him with T. Kezmarsky, a Semmelweis trainee.[21]

Final Descent

Over the years Semmelweis scholars and biographers have offered multiple theories concerning their subject's eccentric personality and the manner in which his final descent occurred, without reaching any consensus. Some have called Semmelweis's mental state an "organic disease of the brain." But such an old-fashioned medical term is so nonspecific that it means next to nothing. It gives no hint as to process. Other biographers, such as Pachner, simply called Semmelweis chronically insane, a term so vague as to be indeterminate. Creutz and Steudel, as well, claimed that he "suffered from chronic insanity for years before his death."[22]

Others described his mental symptoms to be suggestive of manic-depressive illness, most likely without even recognizing such a disease entity. Paul Zweifl, Leipzig professor of obstetrics, declared how very tragic was Semmelweis's insanity: "Later he became so irascible that he was unable to see anybody else's point of view, this state alternating with chronic depression and melancholia."[23] And G. Theodore Gram lamented Semmelweis's "loss of memory and seasons of depression followed by enthusiasm for his conviction." These were "unfortunately the precursors of the disenthronement of a magnificent intellect."[24]

Psychiatrist Istvan Benedek, in his 1967 book *Semmelweis and His Age*, attempted to explain Semmelweis's decline as occurring in three different stages, all mutually interdependent. In the first phase Semmelweis suffered chronically from "psychopathia," a condition that culminated in 1861 but never progressed on to insanity. Benedek considered the second phase a "chronic degeneration of the nervous system," most likely neurosyphilis. This state "progressed in gradual stages from 1861 onwards and became acute in the summer of 1865." Finally, Benedek saw the third phase as an "acute infectious mental disturbance" secondary to osteomyelitis. Death was caused by pyemia.[25] While Hegar is correct regarding Semmelweis's acute infectious decline, the facts regarding his years of eccentric behavior do not at all point to neurosyphilis. Since no evidence, either clinical or pathologic, exists to support a diagnosis of neurosyphilis, it does not warrant further consideration. As discussed below, a diagnosis of chronic manic-depressive illness makes eminent sense. But first, let us consider the mechanisms behind his final, acute decline.

Septic Psychosis

The event that sealed Semmelweis's fate was a recapitulation of Kolletschka's death, the laceration of his finger and contraction of a bacterial infection, followed by a terminal sepsis. With the multiple boils covering his body and an overall course proving less fulminating than that generally seen with streptococcus, Semmelweis most likely succumbed to a staphylococcal infection.

During the final several weeks of his life, Semmelweis suffered from two diseases. Although bipolar disease might explain his years of eccentricities, and even some of his irrational behavior in the latter stages of his life, his acute terminal deterioration cannot be attributed to that disease. His "insanity," as diagnosed by Bokai, was rather a mistaken case of "septic mania" or "septic psychosis," two terms not unheard of in Semmelweis's era. His rapid downward spiral had its onset, at the latest, in late June or early July 1865, beginning with the laceration to his right middle finger, whatever its origin. Subsequent developments point to the laceration as being chronic, an injury sustained approximately four to six weeks prior to his entry into the asylum. Maria's later testimony suggests that the injury had been sustained in early July. But it is known that his entry examination into the asylum provided "proof" (as documentable as the shoddy record keeping would have allowed) that the laceration existed at the time that he was admitted. By that time it was not only gangrenous, but he had a fever and tachycardia, as well. The skin overlying his cut was "reactive," something that takes days, at a minimum, to develop.

Toxic Encephalopathy

With the more refined methods for recognizing and treating such ailments in the modern day, the term "septic mania" is more appropriately called "toxic encephalopathy." The most likely scenario explaining Semmelweis's demise would have begun with the finger laceration in the early days of July. As self-treatment failed, the wound infection worsened, soon followed by reaction of the skin overlying the wound. As the wound deteriorated, inflammation spread into the lymphatics and the blood vessels coursing up his arm, reminiscent of the earliest stages of puerperal fever. Next came the osteomyelitis in the elbow (olecranon). Such an infection could have resulted from direct spread, but it is much more likely that the bone infection occurred secondary to seeding of bacteria into the bloodstream, the earliest sign of sepsis. As bacteria invade the bloodstream, they can infect many tissues, including bone. Osteomyelitis which is, in effect, an abscess of bone, requires a minimum of two to four weeks to develop after the onset of sepsis. It would therefore have been moderately well advanced by the time he was admitted to the asylum. Once osteomyelitis becomes established, it serves as an excellent source for chronic, intermittent seeding of bacteria into the circulation. With no definitive treatment available, such as antibiotics, these episodes of bacterial seeding continue uninterrupted until, finally, sepsis becomes irreversible, and death ensues.

The Greek root word for sepsis means literally "putrefaction" of the blood. Although the terms "septic mania" and "septic psychosis" were known in Semmelweis's time, practitioners knew next to nothing about the ongoing process itself. Being ignorant of the role played by bacteria in sepsis, they knew only that some sort of disintegration of blood was taking place but nothing more. In the late nineteenth century, British physician William Hunter developed an interest in the problem, at a time in which focal causes of sepsis ran rampant throughout the populace of all countries. Most cases of chronic, focal sepsis arose from oral sources, such as carious or abscessed teeth, gum disease, infected tonsils, and the like. As Hunter studied the malady further, he became impressed by the extraordinary variety of distant ill effects produced by sepsis. One effect, in particular, that could be manifest under the rubric of focal sepsis was called "neurotoxic."[26] The clinical picture of a distant, neurotoxic effect might run the spectrum of non-specific signs, beginning with irritability, agitation, disorientation, confusion, stupor, and even coma. Or it could even mimic a full-blown psychosis, dominated by irrational behavior with spurts of perfect lucidity.[27] With the advent of antibiotics and better diagnostic techniques, the public face of septic psychosis began to change over the course of time. What had been a ubiquitous malady of the nineteenth century, seen commonly in its "walking" form, slowly evolved into a disease observed mainly in the desperately ill few, those residing in the modern intensive care unit of the twentieth century.

Doctor Cotton

In 1927, Hunter reported on the experiences of a physician known in the literature only as "Doctor Cotton," an employee of a New Jersey mental institution. Although Cotton's study was not tightly controlled, given the era of his study, he began a program of aggressively treating two hundred patients admitted to the facility with psychiatric diagnoses, mainly "psychoses." In those "psychotic" patients in which he also diagnosed a focal septic condition, he carried out the proper surgical treatment for the septic condition, procedures ranging from the drainage of abscesses, tooth extractions, tonsillectomies, and the like, until all signs of focal sepsis had disappeared. Cotton witnessed a dramatic and gratifying reversal of those distant neurotoxic effects in such patients. Some patients, hospitalized as long as two years, experienced a reversal of their "psychoses" within a matter of one or two months. From this experience the term "septic psychosis" became more formally recognized.[28]

Over the ensuing decades, scientists slowly learned much more about the anatomy and physiology of septic psychosis. The brain, being an exquisitely sensitive organ in its normal state, is said to be "immunologically privileged." That is, through a unique anatomic setup, it is protected from almost all metabolic insults suffered by any given patient. The cerebral arteries and the astrocytes, those main cells giving structure to the brain, have a special anatomic relationship that constitutes a metabolic firewall, the "blood-brain barrier." Specialized processes from the astrocytes attach to the vessel walls, making the interface between vessel and brain impenetrable to all circulating molecules that might prove toxic to the sensitive brain tissue. However, if sepsis of a significant severity and duration supervenes, two different events can occur. First, the body goes into a catabolic state, that is, a state that is the direct opposite of the weight lifter consuming anabolic steroids. In sepsis, the catabolic state results in an abnormal breakdown of proteins into a variety of toxic amino acids. The inflammatory white blood cells break down, as well, into toxic "inflammatory" molecules. In short, a multitude of toxic compounds is released into the general circulation.

The second effect of sepsis is exerted directly on the blood-brain barrier. Those fine astrocytic projections that are attached so tightly to the cerebral arteries are slowly broken down by circulating toxins, creating wide defects within the blood-brain barrier, much as some toxic acid might dissolve the grout in between tiles in a shower, rendering it no longer watertight. Now a myriad of toxic molecules, both large and small, can easily enter into that previously immunologically privileged substance of the brain. Once in the brain, the toxic elements exert multiple deleterious effects, principally on neurons and their interconnections. Neurotransmission becomes flawed as serotonin and other transmitters are altered. As the levels of toxic metabolites wax and wane in the substance of the brain, they produce a corresponding variety of waxing and waning human behaviors, ranging from confusion to hallucinations, convulsions to coma, and so on. As confusion and delirium wax stronger, certain coordinated behaviors, which might make sense in one particular setting, are inappropriate when carried out in another. Being disruptive at a dinner party or reading a midwives' oath to fellow faculty members might be but two different manifestations of "toxic encephalopathy." Whether called septic psychosis or toxic encephalopathy, the term depicts a diffuse chemical inflammation within the substance of the brain.

If such sepsis remains untreated, it can have several different forms of expression within the brain, ranging from toxic encephalopathy to meningitis, encephalitis, or abscesses. In Semmelweis's case, toxic encephalopathy constituted the "insanity" as perceived by Bokai. Semmelweis's findings at autopsy, as described by Scheutauer, were consistent with that diagnosis. The brain revealed changes of inflammation throughout, with edema and infiltration of white blood cells throughout its substance. There were no abscesses, no bacterial infiltrates. No changes suggestive of neurosyphilis could be found. Semmelweis's behavior during his terminal several weeks was entirely consistent with septic mania or toxic encephalopathy. No evidence or need therefore exists to invoke diagnoses that others have suggested, including neurosyphilis, hydrocephalus, nonspecific "brain wasting," Alzheimer's disease, or other entities.

Manic-Depressive Illness

In spite of Bokai's contentions, Semmelweis was almost certainly not insane at the time of his abrupt decline. Not only were his periods of irrationality episodic rather than sustained, but he was completely rational much, if not most, of the time. In his final days, he even participated in his own treatment plans. His chronically abnormal moods, whether characterized by anger, irritability, mania, or depression, generally cycled in a manner more consistent with manic-depressive illness rather than an ongoing psychosis.

Manic-depressive illness, although unrecognized and undiagnosed for his entire life, was responsible for his many years of eccentricity, anger, depression, and paranoia. Excluding perhaps some psychotherapeutic role played by a clinician, if Semmelweis's bipolar disease could not be recognized, clearly it remained untreated. Even if the disease had been diagnosable, lithium, the definitive medication for treating manic-depressive illness, was unavailable until the early 1980s. Other drugs, such as antipsychotics, antidepressants, and anticonvulsants, used more on an adjuvant basis, became available only a few decades before lithium. It is therefore not surprising that Semmelweis's moods slowly worsened with time. The natural course of his disease played out over many years subject to the vicissitudes of his stressful life. American psychology professor David J. Miklowitz cites environmental stressors, or "life events stress," as powerful determinants on the course of bipolar disorder.

Patients with high stress levels have a four to five times greater likelihood of experiencing relapses when compared to those with low to medium life events stress scores.[29] Clearly, Semmelweis lived with high stress throughout his professional career. While it likely exacerbated the course of his disease over the three to four decades of his career, it accounted, as well, for his flamboyantly irrational episodes during the latter stages of his working life. However, he was, for the most part, rational until the end—until sepsis rendered him confused and irrational.

During his major literary efforts with *Aetiology* and *Letters*, Semmelweis was likely in a sustained hypomania, if not a full-blown mania. Manias are often pleasurable experiences, like the highs one might experience with certain illicit psychotropic drugs. It is common for writers, composers, and other creative individuals suffering from bipolar disorder to produce some of their most creative works during such times. In her book *Touched with Fire*, a work relating creativity to manic-depressive illness, Kay Redfield Jamison cites numerous studies that correlate productivity with mania and depression. She points to the highly illustrative case of known manic-depressive composer, Robert Schumann. His two most productive years by far, 1840 and 1849, came during extended periods characterized as hypomanic.[30] When one compares Schumann's number of compositions per year, expressed in bar graph form, they appear as stark and over-towering as two smoke stacks rising from a coal-fired power plant on an otherwise flat desert floor. Although it is a much less frequent phenomenon, some bipolar patients even remain productive through their depressive cycles. In short, Semmelweis's decades of eccentric but productive behavior are entirely consistent with patterns displayed by someone suffering the ravages of manic-depressive illness.

Just as his clinical picture fits the template of manic-depressive illness, so too do his pathologic findings. Biographers and scholars have made much of two different abnormalities found within Semmelweis's brain at autopsy. Most striking was the moderate degree of cerebral atrophy, especially in the frontal lobe regions. In addition, the natural cavities, the ventricles (which hold the cerebrospinal fluid), within Semmelweis's brain were moderately enlarged. Both changes are nonspecific and can be associated with many different conditions, such as advanced age, head injury, hydrocephalus, and degenerative states, including either Alzheimer's or Pick's disease. Some scholars, such as Nuland, Heger, and Benedek, have used these findings to support their contentions that Semmelweis suffered specifically from such ailments as Alzheimer's disease, neurosyphilis, nonspecific dementia, or some other brain disease.

But these findings within Semmelweis's brain are just as consistent with one who has suffered from manic-depressive psychosis for many years, a condition from which Semmelweis was clearly a victim. Modern research into manic-depressive illness lends additional support to the contention that Semmelweis's brain findings are consistent with manic-depressive illness. As detailed in Goodwin's and Jamison's superb work of 2008, *Manic-Depressive Illness: Bipolar Disorders and Recurrent Depression*, newer studies using computerized tomography and magnetic resonance imaging of the human brain have shed new light on changes wrought on cerebral tissue by manic-depressive illness. On multiple occasions, investigators structured such studies, carried out in the 1980s and 1990s, in a manner that allowed for the accurate quantitation of brain mass in patients suffering from bipolar disease. They scanned, as well, normal patients who served as "healthy controls." As a result, researchers were able to determine that patients with bipolar disease exhibited significant wasting in critical regions, mainly at the base of the brain and in the medial frontal regions. Such brain wasting causes a concomitant "passive" increase in volume of the cerebral ventricles, as well as "cortical sulcal enlargement," otherwise known as cortical atrophy (atrophy of white and/or gray matter).[31]

Such changes are similar to the autopsy findings that Scheutauer encountered in Semmelweis's brain. Although Semmelweis's frontal atrophy was more extensive, twenty years of untreated illness and continued stresses might account for more widespread changes. It is certainly more tenable to attribute these autopsy findings to the manic-depressive illness from which Semmelweis had been suffering for decades than it is to merely attribute them blindly to miscellaneous conditions, such as Alzheimer's disease, neurosyphilis, and other neurodegenerative conditions, for which there is no other supporting evidence.

Subsequent experimental imaging studies demonstrate that severe stress causes demonstrable changes in cerebral tissues. Continued repeated experimental stress inflicted on nonhuman subjects causes a loss of the robust interconnections between neurons (dendritic arborizations) in the same critical parts of the nervous system as mentioned above.[32] Although the studies are in nonhumans, they add further evidence that mental stress, such as that seen in manic-depressive illness, is detrimental to the normal trophic health of cerebral tissue.

But these discoveries, since they demonstrate a nonspecific wasting of brain tissue, prohibit one from drawing conclusions that are specific to any one particular disease. Of even more significance are some specific and positive changes observed in the brain in an elegant 2002 radiological imaging study by Gould and Manji, a study that factored lithium into their experimental scheme. This group performed three-dimensional magnetic resonance imaging studies structured in the aforementioned way that allowed them to quantitate brain tissue volumes. First, they scanned patients suffering from bipolar disease at baseline—medication free for two weeks. The same patients were then rescanned after four weeks of lithium treatment maintained at therapeutic levels. Gould and Manji discovered that chronic lithium treatment significantly increased total gray matter content within the brain, while not affecting white matter volume. While one cannot make sweeping conclusions from a single study, it does suggest that therapeutic levels of lithium increases brain mass by reversing at least one form of cerebral "wasting" in patients suffering from bipolar disease.[33] Just as cerebral atrophy can lead to a passive enlargement of the ventricles, so too can an increase in total gray matter lead to a concomitant decrease in ventricular size, that is, a reversal of pathologic changes.

Obviously the newer research cited above does not conclusively establish manic-depressive illness as the sole cause of Semmelweis's many years of eccentricities and mood fluctuations. It is, however, the most tenable explanation to date. This argument best unifies all of the prior enigmas, those loose strings dangling around Semmelweis's life story, a situation made worse by a paucity of biographical information in an era bereft of a solid scientific base.

Resurrection

Given the enormity of Semmelweis's discovery, one might speculate that it would be but a short time before his image would undergo a justifiable resurrection. However, for such a development to happen, the world of medical science would have to progress to a higher plane of enlightenment, a level in which the facts surrounding Semmelweis's contentions were so indisputable that the brilliance of his induction could no longer be denied. Some of these signs of improvement had begun even before Semmelweis's death, but they were isolated cases that, even viewed collectively, would do little to swing the pendulum back to a more balanced position. In fact, a movement to improve his image required nearly three decades to reach its full strength.

As early as 1864, August Hirsch, follower and former student of Semmelweis, published a handbook of pathology in which he claimed that the "noxious agents" responsible for puerperal fever may reside in pus and ichorous matter. In other words, any putrescent tissue can cause the disease, not just cadaveric matter. Of course that was nothing new to the *Lehre*, yet his book proved influential enough to help weaken resistance to Semmelweis's theory.[1]

Another of the first signs of change occurred right under the nose of old Semmelweis nemesis, Carl Braun. In 1860, Karl Mayrhofer, Division I assistant at the Vienna lying-in hospital, began a microscopic study of bodily fluids taken from all puerperal fever victims. He soon discovered bacteria, which he called "vibriones," growing in such fluids. He not only concluded that this microscopic life was responsible for puerperal fever, but he also indicted the physician's examining finger as the principle means of transmission.[2] In 1863, when Braun became more fully aware of Mayrhofer's activities and how close his views were to Semmelweis's, he brought his junior's project to an immediate halt by firing him.

Committee of Experts

One notable development of 1863, two years before Semmelweis's death, revealed how resistance to the theory was slowly crumbling. Austrian authorities, planning a new maternity hospital in Prague, formed a committee of eminent medical men, including Rokitansky and Skoda from Vienna, Virchow from Berlin, as well as some others. Hoping to incorporate the latest information on the cause of puerperal fever into safer construction of their hospital, authorities posed this question to the committee: "According to the present position of science regarding the contagious origin and extension of puerperal fever, is the theory established for certain, is it probable or is it possible?" Rokitansky and Skoda considered its contagious nature "beyond question." Virchow, still mired in theories of "diffuse and malignant inflammation," declared that contagion could only occur at the height of an epidemic. However, Virchow must have finally seen that his was the losing side in this extended debate. By 1864, "the Pope of German Medicine" finally accepted Semmelweis's theory completely.[3] Whether Semmelweis even knew of this eminent conversion, or how it might have affected him, is unknown.

Spaeth

And then there was old Semmelweis adversary, Professor Spaeth, the man who had experienced the wrath of Semmelweis's pen in *Letters*. After his own thorough review of puerperal fever at Vienna General Hospital, he realized that Semmelweis had been correct from the start. In spite of Semmelweis's hotly worded letter to him, Spaeth, in an 1864 article, was professional enough to finally acknowledge publicly that Semmelweis's theory and chloride regimen were correct. Spaeth posed the question: "What consideration then does Semmelweis merit? . . . Certainly, the theory would have gained more obstetricians as open friends, if in the beginning Semmelweis had not represented the facts most obvious to him from one point of view, as the whole, and later defended his theory in a tone which no man of science had been accustomed to up to this time. . . . I also venture to state unreservedly that there is no longer any obstetrician, who is not most deeply convinced of the correctness of Semmelweis' views, even though he may still talk very much against them."[4]

Spaeth must have had Semmelweis's other critic, Scanzoni, in mind as one who still talked against the theory despite being convinced of its correctness. But even Scanzoni's mind had evolved to some extent. In his 1867 *Lehrbuch*, he declared, "We must look upon it as an achievement of recent times that the import of this extremely pernicious . . . malady has been now more exactly determined. . . . Puerperal fever is almost unanimously considered to be an infectious disease." He went on to admit that the disease was a pyemia, or sepsis, "preceded by the admission of products of putrid decomposition of animal matter into the blood-mass."[5] Spaeth finally conceded that contagion came, not from the medium of the atmosphere, but rather from putrid matter on the hands of the practitioner, poorly washed bed linens, and so forth. In essence, he sounded just like Semmelweis, although at no time did he give any recognition to Semmelweis by name.[6]

Following scientific progress chronologically, the next major clinical development occurred in 1865, although it was based upon the obscure work, eight years earlier, of Louis Pasteur. In August 1857, Pasteur, a chemist rather than a physician, delivered an address before the French Academy of Science in which he described a new world of microscopic organisms that he had discovered while working on the fermentation of wines. He asserted that these microorganisms not only existed in various forms, but were also capable of influencing different activities of nature. Each class or type of bacteria had some mysterious power within it to cause the process of fermentation to proceed in different, yet very specific, directions. If fermentation occurred in the proper direction, the desired product, such as wine or cheese, resulted. But, if it proceeded in the wrong direction, a slimy, malodorous waste was the likely product. When Pasteur looked at such ferments under the microscope, he could see that, in the instance of wine, the finished product was associated with one specific bacterial type, whereas the malodorous, wasteful product revealed an abundance of different appearing organisms. It became obvious to him that these microorganisms were in control of this natural process of fermentation. The scientific community was generally skeptical of Pasteur's assertions, and little was made of his address. Pasteur, of course, labored on, publishing his work in an arcane chemistry journal, one read only by those few within the profession. But at least the journal existed in print, free to anyone outside the profession of chemistry who might wish to read it.

Meanwhile, in 1865, thousands of miles away in Glasgow, a general surgeon, Joseph Lister, had been laboring under a fierce load of wound infections in his patients. Widespread infections had been plaguing the medical and surgical wards, not just in Glasgow, but the world over. So withering was his infection rate that Lister had become melancholic over his own inability to combat such conditions with any degree of effectiveness. He could hardly carry out any operation for fear of his patient succumbing to a wound infection. One particularly dangerous condition that he had to face on a near-daily basis was fractures of the extremities. When such fractures were compound, a condition in which bone penetrates the skin, the likelihood of infection progressing to fulminating sepsis and death was very high. Physicians monitored such wounds closely, watching for tissue redness and swelling, the very first signs of incipient infection. So rapid was the deterioration once inflammation set in that surgeons amputated the fractured extremity immediately, in the desperate hope of saving the patient's life.

Then, in August 1865, as Semmelweis lay dying in the Viennese asylum, Lister, quite by accident, came across Pasteur's work in the chemistry journals. After digesting the articles, Lister immediately spotted an analogy between abnormal ferments of wine and wound infections: microscopic life was, on the one hand, controlling and waylaying the wine ferment, while, on the other, invading a wound and producing an abnormal ferment of a different kind, a purulent (pus-filled) wound, rather than one that healed uneventfully. Both were, in essence, infections—one of wine, the other of living tissues.

Using Pasteur's basic scientific work with bacteria as his theoretical foundation, Lister devised his own clinical scientific regimen. If the main source of infection came from microbes in the air, as Pasteur claimed, Lister would work to minimize that danger while allowing the wound to heal. Using carbolic acid as his cleansing agent, he planned to debride (cleanse) the wound and then cover it with a thick, protective dressing impregnated with the same carbolic acid. His initial results—clean, pus-free wounds—lifted his melancholic cloud and energized him to continue onward. Soon he began collecting a series of patients with compound fractures all treated in the same manner, and his results proved stellar. Realizing that his regimen was revolutionary, Lister was off and running, expanding his treatments to patients with abscesses and other forms of infection. In 1867, Lister published his results in a series of articles in two prestigious journals. In the process, he called his prophylactic regimen "antisepsis." Once the effectiveness of his regimen was undeniable, he delivered an address to the British Medical Association that proved epochal: "Since the antiseptic treatment has been brought into full operation, and wounds and abscesses no longer poison the atmosphere with putrid exhalations, my wards . . . have completely changed their character, so that during the last nine months not a single instance of pyaemia, hospital gangrene or erysipelas has occurred in them."[7]

One might think that, once his physician contemporaries had exercised their own due diligence by vetting Lister's method properly, such good news would have spread like wildfire. But such was hardly the case. Despite the obvious clinical benefits of his scheme, Lister still required approximately twenty years of a deliberate and calculated campaign to convince the physicians of Britain and Europe that his antiseptic regimen was valid.

Not only were the general physicians of England slow to adopt Lister's antiseptic regimen, but, in the field of obstetrics, the benefits of antisepsis were even slower to be realized. In fact, England, the country that had led all others in low rates of puerperal fever up to the 1850s, had slipped into a state of chaos. In 1875, in an effort to combat their puerperal fever epidemics and improve their own level of awareness, the Obstetrical Society of London held a great debate on the "Relation of Puerperal Fever to Other Infective Diseases." If the dead can view human proceedings from the other side, Semmelweis would have had a grand time listening as England's most prominent obstetricians pontificated, posing the same questions that Semmelweis had posited to himself and answered correctly nearly thirty years before. Addressing the group, Spencer Wells inquired as to whether anyone had seen "such a case which could not, on careful inquiry, be traced to exposure of the patient to some one or other of the contagious or infectious fevers—to scarlet fever or diphtheria—to measles or smallpox . . .?" What was the value of antiseptics in the prevention and treatment of puerperal fever? Wells then launched into a dissertation on the bacterial research carried out by Pasteur and his observation that germs get their best nutrition from wounds. Bacteria can also enter the blood, effecting "deadly changes in the circulating fluid."[8]

Next, he presented Lister's work and posed the question, "If traumatic fever and pyaemia can be kept out of a surgical hospital why should not puerperal fever be kept out of a lying-in-hospital?"[9] But a number of obstetricians in attendance expressed reservations about this formulation. There was still some unknown aspect to puerperal fever. It was more than a mere local wound fever. Of all speakers, Dr. Graily Hewitt, midwifery professor at University College, came closest to Semmelweis and the truth by calling puerperal fever a blood poisoning—a form of pyemia. The source is an animal poison, which originates from without and is conveyed to the patient by the caregiver—good information, just three decades too late.[10]

Despite all of their work and theorizing concerning puerperal fever, the British had not, as yet, made the precise connection between animal poison and fever. If one became ill through contact with some sort of degenerating animal-organic product, how exactly was the disease conveyed? Louis Pasteur, who had been conducting studies on several women dying of puerperal fever at the Maternité, provided that answer when, in 1860, he first cultured organisms from puerperal fever victims. In that same year, he named the chain-like microbe, the streptococcus.

Yet, progress still proved incredibly slow. In March 1879, nineteen years after discovering the streptococcus, Pasteur attended a meeting of the French Academy of Medicine to hear an address on the subject of puerperal fever by Jacques Hervieux, prominent Parisian accoucheur. Hervieux, who still believed in the spontaneous generation of all life, including bacteria, began by downplaying any potential role that bacteria might play in the origin of puerperal fever.

Bacteria might well be present within a puerperal or surgical wound. However, that did not prove they were the immediate cause of the fever. They were more likely in the wound by coincidence, a mere epiphenomenon. Bacteria arose from within, not from without. The cause, he alleged, was miasmatic air forming as a consequence of all the infections and purulence raging within the hospital. Having finally heard enough of such outdated thinking, Pasteur suddenly found himself up on the stage countering Hervieux and his miasmatic views, delivering a short dissertation on bacteria. Referring to the miasmatic theory, Pasteur stated, "What causes the disease is nothing of the kind; it's the physician and his staff that carry the germ from a sick woman to the healthy one."[11] Drawing the chain of bacteria on the board, Pasteur stated, "There, that is what it is like." During their extended debate, Hervieux remained unconvinced, replying, "I'm afraid I will die before I have seen the microbe [vibrion] that produces this fever."[12] The audience, with views paralleling those of Hervieux, remained skeptical, as well. While it was a notable scene, it proved less than a transformative moment. How could one crude, simple, and invisible microbe explain a disease as complex as puerperal fever?

By this time, 1879, microbial doubters had to admit that bacteria were always present in purulent wounds. But, were they mere epiphenomena, à la Hervieux, or were they the true causative agents, as claimed by bacteriologists? The argument over the role played by bacteria was far from settled, and the road would still prove tortuous. As more years transpired, Pasteur and Robert Koch of Berlin, in particular, would set the science of bacteriology on ever firmer ground. Improved methods for culturing microbes, better bacterial staining techniques employing aniline dyes, and better technology of microscopes all made bacteria that much more vivid, more easily identified, and therefore more believable. Koch better described the multiple types of extant bacteria and even began classifying them by genus and species, just as Linneaus had done for the plant kingdom. As Koch further elucidated diseases, such as anthrax, tuberculosis, cholera, and the like, and identified the bacteria responsible for each disease, it soon became apparent that the natural order was "one specific cause for one specific disease." This was the very idea that Semmelweis had put forth, in cruder form—"decomposed animal organic matter is the *exclusive cause"*—that was deemed so unacceptable by his medical contemporaries. It was Koch, as well, who first uttered the statement that all maladies belonging to the category of "infectious diseases" are the result of bacterial activity.

Koch went even further by creating an algorithm, "Koch's Postulates," to prove how one specific bacterial strain caused one specific disease. In essence, the scheme involved culturing the principle organism from the victim's wound, purifying it by repeated cultures, and then reproducing the disease in another non-human laboratory subject through reinoculation of that purified culture. The final step in this scheme then required recovering that same organism in the second subject through yet one final culture. As Koch, the master bacteriologist, became more celebrated, he held symposia around the world—workshops teaching bacteriological techniques to various and sundry physicians. Pasteur, ever the showman, held public gatherings in which he demonstrated the effectiveness of his specific vaccine in preventing a specific disease. By the mid-1880s, the discipline of bacteriology had metamorphosed from an arcane and viscerally repugnant subject to a vital science with great practical applications. In the minds of scientists and public alike, bacteriology had become an accepted part of the social fabric.

These bacteriological advancements began making Lister's job of proselytizing for antisepsis less difficult, as physicians found his message more credible. By the end of the 1880s, the germ theory was firmly established, and Listerian antisepsis was generally accepted. Its benefits were so obvious that only the most extreme obscurants failed to appreciate its value to mankind. It was only natural that efforts would next progress from antisepsis to the ultimate goal of full asepsis, including the accoutrements of surgical cap, mask, gloves, gown, air purification, and the isolation of infected patients and their pathogenic organisms.

When obstetricians, as a group, finally embraced the practice of antisepsis, they viewed it more as Lister's, rather than Semmelweis's, contribution to the world. A Professor Stadtfelt of Copenhagen had been the first to adopt Lister's regimen back in 1870, well ahead of most other Europeans. His cases of puerperal fever plummeted dramatically, making the benefits of antisepsis undeniable. Most of Europe followed, although it required more than a decade, into the early 1880s, before it was complete. With the dramatic decreases in puerperal morbidity and mortality seen in such centers as London, Paris, Vienna, Boston, and Stockholm, one just had to accept the role that bacteria played in the production of the disease.

General acceptance in Britain and America came even later than on the Continent. It was the mid-1880s before Listerism was fully adopted. By 1888, antisepsis had progressed to the point that London obstetrician, W. S. Playfair, was driven to exclaim: "From being hotbeds of death and disease in which no woman could be confined without serious risk, sometimes hardly less grave than that of a capital surgical operation, in the majority of well-managed lying-in hospitals a woman is now as safe, if not safer, than if she was confined in a large and luxurious private house, with nurse, physician, and all that money can now procure."[13]

Playfair's observation was important because it served as a nidus for Semmelweis's resurrection movement. Then, another obstetrician, Charles Cullingworth, still hoping to convert some of his agnostic colleagues, spoke of the theoretical foundation laid by Pasteur upon which Lister based his work, ultimately bringing a "stupendous revolution in midwifery."[14] Cullingworth fully recognized Semmelweis, albeit belatedly, in an 1888 address "Puerperal Fever: A Preventable Disease." The discovery of the role of bacteria in causing septicemia was the key to the mystery. Now all was accounted for:

> The propagation by personal contact, the manner in which disease dogged the footsteps of individual practitioners, and became the scourge of lying-in hospitals, the fatal results of cadaveric contamination, the deleterious influence of protracted labour, involving, as it did, repeated examinations, the almost entire immunity from the disease of women in the streets and elsewhere, in whom no examination was made, the success that attended the purification of the hands by means of chlorine, all these facts are now easily explained. . . . How much the knowledge of the dependence of septicaemia on micro-organisms, and the methods of treatment founded upon it, have accomplished for surgery, I need not, in this hospital, re-

mind you. What I desire to impress upon you today is, that they are capable of effecting an equally stupendous revolution in midwifery.[15]

Cullingworth's quote, "All these facts are now easily explained," sounded like the ghost of Ignaz Semmelweis, himself explaining to his nescient colleagues the various steps involved in the pathogenesis of puerperal fever some forty-one years earlier. Some physicians were unable to give up on their multifactorial ideas of disease causation. They coped with the new changes wrought by antisepsis by looking the other way as they adopted the preventive regimen. Its benefits could no longer be denied.[16]

In this more receptive atmosphere, Semmelweis's image continued to improve, but the real spark that ignited his resurrection was provided by surgeon Theodore Duka, Hungarian by birth but a naturalized British citizen and follower of Semmelweis's life. In 1886, Duka wrote a two-part article in *Lancet* based upon information gleaned from Jakab Bruck's 1885 biography. He presented Semmelweis as a man "unjustly neglected," promoting a theory that was opposed largely on political grounds. According to Duka, Semmelweis was unable to rise to the challenge with a sufficient level of robustness required to carry on his *Lehre*. The battle made him ultimately "introspective, desponding, irritable and at last unreasonable. He had indomitable industry, a sagacious insight amounting almost to genius, but he had little of the fortitude which enables a man to *labour* and *wait*."[17] Duka's image of Semmelweis morphed into that of the cruelly rejected, genius researcher, prescient savior of young women, a man who wrote a peerless treatise on childbed fever and was driven insane, a martyr to the very disease he had spent his life fighting.

Adding further to the waxing image of Semmelweis as the hero, along with Cullingworth's 1888 address, was influential obstetrician W. E. Fothergill's 1896 book *Manual of Midwifery*. He, too, painted a picture of Semmelweis as a pioneer and "misunderstood martyr."[18]

By the late 1880s, the spirits of British obstetricians had been lifted and reenergized by the successes of Lister. But as they studied the topic further, the work that Semmelweis had carried out some four decades earlier resonated strongly with them. Lister's antiseptic scheme was not all that different from what Semmelweis had proposed more than thirty years before.

The group was struck with a collective guilty conscience. No doubt, Semmelweis had been treated poorly.

British obstetricians decided to make amends. Spencer Wells took the initiative by convening a preliminary committee meeting in his London home in October 1892. In hopes of righting the wrongs perpetrated on Semmelweis decades earlier, they planned to create some sort of memorial to the man. Present at the meeting were W. S. Playfair, Spencer Wells, Joseph Lister, Theodore Duka, and Grailly Hewitt, as well as men known only as Drs. Glover, Bloch, Boxall, and Priestly. With time, this cohort of men joined with the local Budapest Committee, headed by Gustav Dirner, to form the International Semmelweis Memorial Committee.[19] The committee contacted the famous Hungarian sculptor, Alajos Stróbl, who, in 1904, had just completed the soon-to-be iconic Matthias Fountain at Buda Castle. Strobl was commissioned to erect a statue of Semmelweis befitting his new celebrated status.

Finally, on September 30, 1906, in a ceremony that included Maria Semmelweis and a host of international dignitaries, Semmelweis's likeness (fig. 23) was unveiled at the entrance to St. Rochus Hospital in Budapest, where it still stands today. Theodore Duka attended as the British representative.[20] In one memorial speech, Otto Pertik, professor of pathology in Budapest, referred to the reason for Semmelweis's tragedy, "his insanity, was mainly due to the strain of knowing himself in the right and not being able to convince others of it." It caused the "final collapse of his moral order."[21] Gustav Dirner summed up the sentiment of the occasion regarding Semmelweis: "We know today that he belongs to us, and we knew it before too, but for a time—let us be quite frank about this—we had forgotten him completely. Did anybody hear the name of Semmelweis as much as mentioned in a university lecture throughout the seventies, or in the early eighties? Did anybody see his picture, his frowning brow, his searching eyes exhibited anywhere where it could have impressed the susceptible minds of the young generation of doctors? I have not heard his name nor seen his picture even when Lister's teachings reached us and the fume of the carbolic spray made a curtain around the bed of the laboring woman. But at long

last his name is heard again."[22] Through the efforts of the Semmelweis Committee, the first steps toward ameliorating the injustice
perpetrated upon this tortured man had been accomplished.

Despite some prolonged hiatuses, more long range plans continued. In 1963, Semmelweis's remains at Budapest's Kerepesi Cemetery were disinterred once again and laid to rest for the third time
in a special crypt in the courtyard behind his Taban birth home—
the soon-to-be Semmelweis Museum of Medical History. In 1964,
conversion of the museum was completed. Next were plans for a
medical library. The Hungarian Library of Medicine, a research facility, had existed for many years in differing iterations and loca-
tions. Finally, in 1968, it coalesced into one site, on the Buda side of
the Danube, as the Semmelweis Medical Library, named in honor of
Hungary's most notable man of medicine.

Semmelweis remained a celebrated figure throughout the twentieth century with virtually no one, except perhaps Loudon, challenging his unique status as an international icon of medical science.
That is, until 2003, when the late Dr. Sherwin B. Nuland, medical
historian and noted Semmelweis scholar, published *The Doctors'
Plague*, a biography in which he challenged the "mythic" image of
Semmelweis as the great icon of medicine. In Nuland's view, the
pendulum of Semmelweis adulation had swung too far—resurrecting
his image from a life of near-ignominy to one of unwarranted idola-
try. Nuland, echoing some of the same charges as Loudon, claimed
that virtually all biographies written in the first sixty years of the
twentieth century have amounted to hagiographies by writers still
caught up in the imagery evoked by Duka, Waldheim, and English
obstetricians such as Fothergill.[23] They viewed Semmelweis's life
as a tragedy "in the manner of Aeschylus, in which the hero is destroyed by malevolent gods—by forces beyond his control." But Nuland contended that Semmelweis's life had more in common with a
Sophoclean tragedy in which the hero was propelled to a tragic end
more by faults within his own personality than by any influences by
the gods.[24] Few would argue that point.

Nuland objected to the common biographic image of Semmelweis "fighting a lonely battle against the ignorance and arrogance
of authority, as though the entire established hierarchy of mid-19th
century medicine had arrayed itself against him."[25] According to

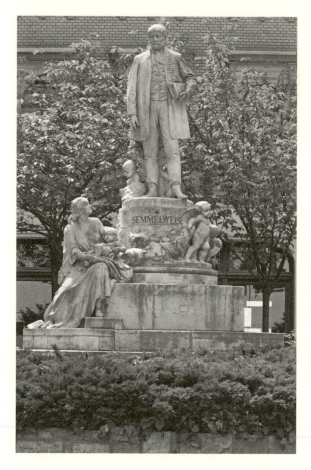

Figure 23. Commemorative statue of Ignaz Semmelweis sculpted by Alajos Stróbl (1856–1926) in 1906
and standing today at the entrance to Saint Rochus
Hospital in Budapest. Photograph by Theodore G.
Obenchain.

this scenario, only Semmelweis understood the great truth being
offered to the world. Of course, that was the case. Virtually no one
understood the nuanced shades of his *Lehre*, let alone his idea of
exclusivity. Nuland went on to state that Semmelweis's theory represented such a great threat to members of the power structure that
they conspired to defeat him. Authorities not only forced the man to
leave Vienna, they even drove him insane. In the final scene of this
tragedy, according to Nuland, Semmelweis succumbed to the very

disease that he had been fighting against so courageously throughout his life. "It provided the narrative of his life's journey with the
final dramatic moment that would make it an epic saga," he wrote.[26]

But, as Nuland asserted, it was Semmelweis himself who was the
main person responsible for the tragic events in his life. He entered
the battle with too many strikes against him, his defeat preordained.
Semmelweis retreated to the "protective cocoon" of Pest, "an intellectual backwater," because he could not compete in the elegant
environment of imperial Vienna: "The drama of Ignaz Semmelweis
lies in the fact that, just as he discovered his own truth and his own
mission, he created and impelled himself toward his own tragic des-
tiny. This is precisely how Sophocles might have written it, with a
Greek chorus of dying mothers—a great hero, a great truth, a great
mission, and finally, a mad flight of passionate arrogance resulting
in destruction. The gods who were the professors of obstetrics did
not bring it about; the hero brought it on himself."[27]

In my opinion, Nuland judged Semmelweis too harshly, while
letting the professors of obstetrics off too easily. Semmelweis was
fighting a lonely and losing battle against the ignorance and arrogance of established authority. But the larger question is whether or
not Semmelweis "brought it on himself." Nuland appears to have
believed that Semmelweis was little more than a curmudgeon, an
ill-tempered and angry man, but one whose psychological profile
still fell within gross limits of normal, until Alzheimer's disease
supervened, bringing about his premature and tragic end. In other
words, he suffered, at worst, from a chronic, non-specific type of
mental aberration, much like some village crank. Nuland discount-
ed the repressive atmosphere of Viennese medical culture, the tensions between Old and New School, and the shameful manner in
which imperial authorities had dealt with its prior medical pioneers.
In that context, Semmelweis's decision was not all that unreasonable, although the isolated manner in which he carried it out was
peculiar. Nuland leveled other charges; that Semmelweis was, by
choice, a solitary figure in a lonely quest, deliberately shunning
those around him; that he was, in effect, negligent for failing to utilize the microscope in his research, and so on.[28]

As I read such critical comments early in my research, I became
determined to answer each of Nuland's unreasonable strikes against

Semmelweis, point by detailed point. But, as I became more deeply involved in the subject of Semmelweis, the more insights I gained into his psyche. This was not just some eccentric miscreant. He was suffering the effects of at least three decades of manic-depressive illness. His mania became evident when he began writing *Aetiology*. But that was only half of the picture. His bouts of depression, his angry confrontations, his lugubrious moods, and his eccentricities point to a more generalized and pernicious problem with his personality. With the exception of Sillo-Seidl, whose book was published in 1978, no one, including Nuland, appeared to have any idea that the man was suffering from manic-depressive illness. It is not that Nuland grossly underestimated the debilitating role bipolar disease played during the three decades of Semmelweis's career; he was completely unaware of its presence. It is that lack of awareness of the major driving force in Semmelweis's life that I believe minimizes Nuland's points of argumentation and renders them both moot and superfluous. The long-term effects of Semmelweis's mental illness were a major determinant of his journey through life, as much as, if not more than, were his deliberate, willful acts. These two forces cannot be separated. Therefore, Nuland's points of argumentation, the majority with which I generally disagree, can be largely dismissed as outmoded.

Part of Semmelweis's personality and the changes that began somewhere in the 1850s—his imbalanced life, his over-devotion to work in a depressing environment with no vacation in nearly twenty years, seem significant psychologically. He deteriorated from a young and happy social being into an asocial obsessive pursuing his medical theory in solitude.[29] How much was wrought by his imposed work schedule, and how much was an early manifestation of his manic-depressive illness is impossible to say. But clearly he was a victim of his heredity and the behavioral changes already preprogrammed into his DNA. Certain facets of one's personality, such as paranoia, suspiciousness, obsessiveness, excessive anger, and so on, shaped and exacerbated by life's stressors, emerge over time according to their own preordained schedules.

Semmelweis had to contend with two adversaries, the first of which was his manic-depressive disease. Second were the antiquated state of medical theory and the general failure of the leaders of medical science to break through their bonds of medievalism. Their resistance provided a background of continuing social stresses to Semmelweis that kept him filled with anger and resentment through most of his career. What little proselytizing Semmelweis did, he was forced to preach to the only crowd available, a complacent, chauvinistic, and sometimes ignorant group of physicians who either refused to vet his theory objectively or to reexamine their own primitive level of enlightenment. As noted scientist and writer Carl Sagan observed: "At the heart of science is an essential balance between two seemingly contradictory attitudes—an openness to new ideas, no matter how bizarre or counterintuitive they may be, and the most ruthless skeptical scrutiny of all ideas, old and new. This is how deep truths are winnowed from deep nonsense."[30] In other words, scientific idealism should be counterbalanced by "ruthless scrutiny," rather than slothful ignorance. In the middle of nineteenth-century Vienna, Ignaz Semmelweis offered the world a new and deep truth concerning contagion, only to have it rejected. The greater medical community of Austria had benefitted from multiple presentations of that theory by such luminaries as Hebra and Skoda. Semmelweis himself had even spelled out the points of his theory distinctly. His follow-up argument, *Aetiology* and *Letters*, may have been circumlocutory, bombastic, even repugnant in style, yet both were still cogent and well-reasoned arguments. It was the professors and the medical community that failed to furnish that counterbalance of unbiased, rational scrutiny, creating a tension that would dog Semmelweis for the rest of his life.

Semmelweis may have acquired a reputation of being perpetually angry, misanthropic, and an "eccentric faddist." He may have even been plagued by some level of "chronic insanity," yet he carried on a full load of work until the very end—hardly the actions of one who is overtly insane. Another indicator of the soundness of his mind concerned his ability to compartmentalize important factors when he deemed it appropriate. He could be selectively "misanthropic" to those he considered dishonest or intellectually slothful, and to those hospital staff members who employed passive aggressive methods against him and his regimen. But the manner in which he treated those beneath him provided a more accurate insight as to his mental condition. Medical students, and a few cooperative nursing staff members, both liked and respected Semmelweis. No one had a better insight than they as to how devoted, how sincere, and how right he was. The relationship Semmelweis had with his patients and the poor provided an even better insight into his sanity. He remained unwaveringly kind and gentle to them all until the very end, when toxic encephalopathy supervened.

Nuland also asserted that Semmelweis probably died as a result of Alzheimer's disease. But no clinical evidence exists to support such a notion. Semmelweis's mental changes late in life resembled a psychosis more than a dementia. While he was not psychotic, Semmelweis was even further from being demented. Since Alois Alzheimer did not even describe the unique changes in the brain until 1901, nineteenth-century pathologists could not look to the microscopic exam of his brain for the diagnosis. Up until Semmelweis's fateful speech to the faculty, marking the beginning of his final descent, he had been active in running a university department, had just published an article on ovariotomy, and was authoring a textbook on obstetrics—hardly the picture of a man with a chronic, progressively debilitating disease like Alzheimer's. Even in his final two weeks, when he suffered from toxic encephalopathy, he had, at a minimum, significant periods of lucidity.

But Nuland's most serious misjudgment of his subject cannot be attributed to his failure to recognize the presence of bipolar disease. He considered it ironic how Semmelweis could be lionized as an icon of medicine when he had exerted "no lasting effect" on obstetrics.[31] He had not even been "a herald of the oncoming order."[32] But, as Professor Codell Carter pointed out in 1981, "Semmelweis was very likely the first to identify a single and necessary cause for all cases of a particular disease and to recharacterize the disease in terms of that necessary cause."[33] Coming from a man who was not only forced to contend with the orthodox world of multifactorialism, but who also was, along with the rest of humanity, completely ignorant of microbes and their significance in the natural world, Semmelweis's brilliant inductive leap marked the beginning of modernism. Once the role that bacteria played in disease causation had been elucidated, the concept of "one agent per single disease" was much easier to accept. Semmelweis's theory of infection just happened to be decades ahead of its time. Nuland blithely overlooked this epochal contribution of exclusivity—one specific cause for one specific disease—a concept that proved even too far advanced for Semmelweis's pioneering mentors, Hebra, Skoda, and Rokitansky, to fathom.

Semmelweis offered the concept of exclusivity to the world of medicine, even though the tyrannical majority rejected it during his lifetime. Like a Cassandra, he stood resolutely by his idea, even as he was surrounded for so many years by the doubting multifactorialists. That, alone, is extraordinary. But, remarkably, Semmelweis's idea of single and necessary in the context of disease causation has withstood the test of 160 years—his language refined somewhat, but still as fundamentally correct today as it was in 1847. To state that Semmelweis had not even been "a herald of the oncoming order" while ignoring that glaring fact is inaccurate and unfair.

Ignaz Semmelweis was a martyr to the world of human foibles.[34] As one considers the entire spectrum of human vices, ranging from anger, cowardice, envy, pride, greed, vanity, sloth, and jealousy, each played some contributory role in producing one of the greatest tragic figures in all the history of medical science. Clearly Semmelweis's poor communication skills combined with his odd personality and bipolar disease rendered him a flawed leader of a revolution. Yet, he dedicated his life to the victims of puerperal fever, never resting in his goal to solve this devastating disease while exposing the world to a new age of scientific medicine, all while being tragically frustrated by an unreceptive medical community.

Since it was only posthumously that Semmelweis gained recognition for his epic discovery, one has to take a long view of history in order to agree with Bruck's heartening conclusion regarding the man: "We deplore his martyrdom, but we can find some comfort in the reflection, that he did not struggle in vain, and that he did not suffer in vain. The whole civilized world was soon to enjoy the fruits of his immeasurably beneficent discovery. He had thrown the light of scientific progress into a region hitherto shrouded in the darkness of Egyptian night."[35]

Whether or not Semmelweis struggled or suffered in vain, he would have been heartened, his pains ablated, were he able to view the scientific progress leading to the elucidation of the role of bacteria in puerperal fever. The essence of his "toxic particles" turned out to be microscopic life—invisible entities that proved both sufficient and necessary in causing diseases. These facts not only vindicated his entire effort, but they also led, eventually, to his resurrection. The role that microscopic life played in puerperal fever specifically, and in nature generally, was at long last revealed and broadly accepted. Ultimately, this led to the fulfillment of Semmelweis's prophetic thoughts expressed at the youthful age of forty-two in his epilogue to *Aetiology*: "If I look back into the past with my present conviction, then I can banish the melancholy which overtakes me, looking at the same time into that happy future, in which within and without the lying-in hospitals over the entire world only cases of auto-infection will occur. . . . But should it not be given to me, which God forbid, to behold this happy time with my own eyes, the conviction that this time will come without fail sooner or later after me, will soothe the hour of my death."[36]

Notes

Introduction

1. W. Campbell, "On Puerperal Fever," *London Medical Gazette* 9 (1831–32): 353–54, cited in Irvine Loudon, *The Tragedy of Childbed Fever* (Oxford: Oxford University Press, 2000), 45–46.

2. Loudon, *Tragedy*, 354.

3. Lewis Thomas, *The Youngest Scientist; Notes of a Medical Watcher* (New York: Penguin Books, 1983).

4. Max Planck, *A Scientific Autobiography and Other Papers* (New York: Philosophical Library, 1949), 33–34.

Puerperal Fever

1. J. F. Hervieux, *Traité clinique et pratique des maladies puerperales*, trans. I. Loudon (Paris: 1880), cited in Thomas Dormandy, *Moments of Truth: Four Creators of Modern Medicine* (Chichester: John Wiley and Sons, 2003), 163–64.

2. Loudon, *Tragedy*, 59.

3. John D. Thompson and Grace Goldin, *The Hospital: A Social and Architectural History* (New Haven: Yale University Press, 1975).

4. Ignaz Semmelweis, *The Etiology, the Concept and the Prophylaxis of Childbed Fever*, trans. Frank P. Murphy, with *Open Letters*, trans. Sherwin B. Nuland and Ferenc A. Gyorgyey, The Classics of Surgery Library Special Edition (New York: Gryphon Editions, 1994), 757.

5. Semmelweis, *Etiology*, 757.

6. Semmelweis, *Etiology*, 757–59.

7. Semmelweis, *Etiology*, 759–60.

8. Dieter Jetter, *Geschichte des Hospitals*, vol. 1 (Weisbaden: F. Steiner, 1966), 145.

9. Loudon, *Tragedy*, 6.

10. Loudon, *Tragedy*, 62.

11. Loudon, *Tragedy*, 8.

12. Loudon, *Tragedy*, 6.

13. Charles D. Meigs, *Females and Their Diseases; A Series of Letters to His Class* (Philadelphia: Lea and Blanchard, 1848), 576, accessed March 16, 2014, https://books.google.com/books?id=qOMRAAAAYAAJ&print-sec=frontcover&dq=Females+and+Their+Diseases;+A+Series+of+Let-ters+to+His+Class&hl=en&sa=X&ved=0CB0Q6AEwAGoVChMIur2iy-dyNyQIVhkgmCh0-Zw5c#v=onepage&q=Females%20and%20Their%20Diseases%3B%20A%20Series%20of%20Letters%20to%20His%20Class&f=false.

Prodrome

1. William Sinclair, *Semmelweis: His Life and His Doctrine* (Manches-ter: Manchester University Press, 1909), 8.
2. Georg Sillo-Seidl, *Die Wahrheit uber Semmelweis: Eine Bild-Biogra-phie*, trans. Lori Schultheis (Genf: Ariston Verlag, 1978), 34.
3. K. Codell Carter and Barbara Carter, *Childbed Fever: A Scientific Bi-ography of Ignaz Semmelweis* (Westport, CT: Greenwood Press , 1994), 44.
4. Sinclair, *Semmelweis*, 8.
5. Sinclair, *Semmelweis*, 7–8.
6. Thomas Dormandy, *Moments of Truth: Four Creators of Modern Med-icine* (Chichester: John Wiley and Sons, 2003), 141.
7. Dormandy, *Moments of Truth*, 156.
8. James J. Garber, *Harmony and Healing: The Theoretical Basis for Ancient and Medieval Medicine* (New Brunswick: Transaction Publishers, 2008), 17–18.
9. R. R. Trail, "Sydenham's Impact on English Medicine," *Medical His-tory 9*, no. 4 (October 1965): 356, accessed November 13, 2015, http://www.ncbi.nlm.nih.gov/pmc/articles/PMC1033532/.
10. R. M. Yost, "Sydenham's Philosophy of Science," *Osiris 9* (1950): 91.
11. Trail, "Sydenham's Impact," 359.
12. Kenneth Dewhurst, *Doctor Thomas Sydenham: 1624–1689* (Berke-ley: University of California Press, 1966), 59.
13. Trail, "Sydenham's Impact," 360.
14. Yost, "Sydenham's Philosophy," 98.
15. Yost, "Sydenham's Philosophy," 57.
16. H. M. Sinclair, "Some Ups and Downs of Oxford Science," *Oxford Medicine: Essays on the Evolution of the Oxford Clinical School to Com-memorate the Bicentenary of the Radcliffe Infirmary 1770–1970*, ed. Ken-neth Dewhurst (Oxford: Sandford Publications, 1970), 6.
17. Sinclair, "Some Ups and Downs," 6.
18. Yost, "Sydenham's Philosophy," 103.
19. Yost, "Sydenham's Philosophy," 104.
20. Erna Lesky, *The Vienna Medical School of the 19th Century* (Balti-more: The Johns Hopkins University Press, 1976), 22.
21. Lesky, *Vienna Medical*, 9.
22. Lesky, *Vienna Medical*, 7, 11.
23. Lesky, *Vienna Medical*, 12, 18.
24. Lesky, *Vienna Medical*, 26.

25. Meigs, *Females and Their Diseases*, 580.
26. Lesky, *Vienna Medical*, 23–25.

Old School; New School

1. Lesky, *Vienna Medical*, 107.
2. E. Ashworth Underwood, *Boerhaave's Men: At Leyden and After* (Edinburgh: Edinburgh University Press, 1977), 7–8.
3. Herman Boerhaave, *Aphorisms Concerning the Knowledge and Cure of Diseases*, trans. J. Del Acoste (London: B. Cowsend and W. Innys, 1715), accessed December 22, 2014, https://archive.org/details/boerhaavesaphor-00delagoog.
4. Lesky, *Vienna Medical*, 78.
5. Lesky, *Vienna Medical*, 107.
6. Lesky, *Vienna Medical*, 106.
7. Ralph H. Major, *A History of Medicine*, Vol. 2 (Springfield: Charles C. Thomas, 1954), 782.
8. Lesky, *Vienna Medical*, 108.
9. Lesky, *Vienna Medical*, 120.
10. Josef Skoda, *A Treatise on Percussion and Auscultation*, trans. W. O. Markham, 4th ed. (London: Highly and Son, 1853), 346.
11. Lesky, *Vienna Medical*, 120.
12. Lesky, *Vienna Medical*, 118.
13. Lesky, *Vienna Medical*, 119–20.
14. Lesky, *Vienna Medical*, 121.
15. Dormandy, *Moments of Truth*, 144.
16. Dormandy, *Moments of Truth*, 146.
17. Lesky, *Vienna Medical*, 130–31.
18. Lesky, *Vienna Medical*, 132.
19. Major, *History of Medicine*, 783.
20. Lesky, *Vienna Medical*, 131.
21. Ibid.

Vienna General Hospital

1. Sinclair, *Semmelweis*, 11.
2. Semmelweis, *Etiology*, 355.
3. Dormandy, *Moments of Truth*, 156.
4. Semmelweis, *Etiology*, xlvi.
5. Semmelweis, *Etiology*, xlvi.
6. Lesky, *Vienna Medical*, 54.
7. Sherwin B. Nuland, *The Doctors' Plague: Germs, Childbed Fever, and the Strange Story of Ignac Semmelweis* (New York: W. W. Norton Company, 2003), 103.
8. Lesky, *Vienna Medical*, 55.
9. Dormandy, *Moments of Truth*, 59.
10. Lesky, *Vienna Medical*, 57.
11. Carter and Carter, *Childbed Fever*, 22.

12. Ignaz Semmelweis, *The Etiology, Concept, and Prophylaxis of Childbed Fever*, trans. Codell Carter (Madison: University of Wisconsin Press, 1983), 70.

13. Sinclair, *Semmelweis*, 41.

14. Sinclair, *Semmelweis*, 40–43.

15. Sinclair, *Semmelweis*, 43.

16. Loudon, *Tragedy*, 98.

17. Loudon, *Tragedy*, 94–95.

Puerperal Fever Theories

1. Ferenc A. Gyorgyey, *Puerperal Fever 1847–1861: From the First Statement about the Discovery to the Publication of Semmelweis's Aetiology* (Master's thesis, Yale University, 1968), 44–45.

2. Sinclair, *Semmelweis*, 37–39.

3. Sophia Jex-Blake, "Puerperal Fever: An Inquiry into its Nature and Treatment" (M.D. diss., University of Bern, 1877), 1, cited in Carter and Carter, *Childbed Fever*, 31.

4. Loudon, *Tragedy*, 18.

5. Loudon, *Tragedy*, 19–21.

6. Loudon, *Tragedy*, 29.

7. Frank G. Slaughter, *Immortal Magyar* (New York: Henry Schuman, 1950), 37.

8. Loudon, *Tragedy*, 30–31.

9. Loudon, *Tragedy*, 85.

10. Loudon, *Tragedy*, 11.

11. Herman Tillmanns, *Textbook of Surgery* (New York: D. Appleton and Company, 1901), 347.

12. Slaughter, *Immortal Magyar*, 39.

13. Theodore G. Obenchain, *The Victorian Vivisection Debate: Frances Power Cobbe, Experimental Science and the "Claims of Brutes"* (Jefferson, NC: McFarland and Company, Inc., 2012), 50–51.

Assistantship

1. Sillo-Seidl, *Wahrheit*, 38.

2. Ibid.

3. Gyorgy Gortvay and Imre Zoltan, *Semmelweis: His Life and Work* (Budapest, Hungary: Akademiai Kiado, 1968), 40.

4. Gortvay and Zoltan, *Semmelweis*, 48.

5. Sillo-Seidl, *Wahrheit*, 66.

6. Semmelweis, *Etiology*, xlvi–vii.

7. Slaughter, *Immortal Magyar*, 49.

8. Gortvay and Zoltan, *Semmelweis*, 48.

9. Gyorgy Marikovsky, ed., *Selected Works of Lajos Markusovsky* (Budapest: Magyar Orvosi Konyvkiado Tarsulat, 1905), 27, cited in Gortvay and Zoltan, *Semmelweis*, 48.

10. Gortvay and Zoltan, *Semmelweis*, 39.

11. Gortvay and Zoltan, *Semmelweis*, 50.
12. Dormandy, *Moment of Truth*, 188.
13. Lesky, *Vienna Medical*, 183.

Enlightenment

1. Semmelweis, *Etiology*, 391.
2. Semmelweis, *Etiology*, 390–93.
3. Sinclair, *Semmelweis*, 49.
4. Gortvay and Zoltan, *Semmelweis*, 51.
5. Gortvay and Zoltan, *Semmelweis*, 52.
6. Gortvay and Zoltan, *Semmelweis*, 58.
7. Semmelweis, *Etiology*, 392–93.
8. Semmelweis, *Etiology*, 393–96.
9. Semmelweis, *Etiology*, trans. Carter, 29.
10. Semmelweis, *Etiology*, 395–96.
11. Sinclair, *Semmelweis*, 204.
12. Sinclair, *Semmelweis*, 8.
13. Gortvay and Zoltan, *Semmelweis*, 59.
14. Semmelweis, *Etiology*, xlviii.
15. Gortvay and Zoltan, *Semmelweis*, 74.
16. Gortvay and Zoltan, *Semmelweis*, 60.

Revolution

1. Gortvay and Zoltan, *Semmelweis*, 63.
2. John Merriman, *A History of Modern Europe: From the Renaissance to the Present* (New York: W. W. Norton and Company, 2010), 141.
3. Merriman, *History*, 13–21.
4. Gortvay and Zoltan, *Semmelweis*, 62–63.
5. Merriman, *History*, 141–42.
6. John Merriman and Jay Winter, *Europe 1789 to 1914: Encyclopedia of the Age of Industry and Empire*, Vol. I (Detroit: Thompson Gale, 2006), 634–40.
7. Sinclair, *Semmelweis*, 85.
8. Lesky, *Vienna Medical*, 186.
9. K. Codell Carter and George S. Tate, "Josef Skoda's Relationship to the Work of Ignaz Semmelweis," *Medizin Historisches Journal* 19 (1984): 340.
10. Carter and Tate, "Josef Skoda," 345.
11. Lesky, *Vienna Medical*, 186.
12. Sinclair, *Semmelweis*, 60–70.
13. Semmelweis, *Etiology*, xlviii–xlix.
14. Sinclair, *Semmelweis*, 83.
15. Gortvay and Zoltan, *Semmelweis*, 64.
16. Carter and Tate, "Josef Skoda," 345.
17. Sinclair, *Semmelweis*, 91–92.
18. Gortvay and Zoltan, *Semmelweis*, 68.
19. Sinclair, *Semmelweis*, 94.

20. Sinclair, *Semmelweis*, 97.
21. Sinclair, *Semmelweis*, 98–99.
22. Sinclair, *Semmelweis*, 100.
23. Lesky, *Vienna Medical*, 187.

Semmelweis Speaks

1. Gortvay and Zoltan, *Semmelweis*, 65.
2. Gortvay and Zoltan, *Semmelweis*, 65.
3. Gortvay and Zoltan, *Semmelweis*, 68.
4. Sinclair, *Semmelweis*, 103.
5. Sinclair, *Semmelweis*, 101.
6. Ibid.
7. Gortvay and Zoltan, *Semmelweis*, 69.
8. Sinclair, *Semmelweis*, 109–10.
9. Slaughter, *Immortal Magyar*, 123.
10. Sinclair, *Semmelweis*, 102–3.
11. Lesky, *Vienna Medical*, 187.
12. William Shakespeare, *The Merchant of Venice*, act 2, scene 2, accessed December 23, 2014, http://www.opensourceshakespeare.org/.
13. Lesky, *Vienna Medical*, 187.
14. Loudon, *Tragedy*, 102.
15. Gortvay and Zoltan, *Semmelweis*, 66.
16. Ibid.

Budapest

1. Sinclair, *Semmelweis*, 113–14.
2. Lajos Markusovsky, "Reviewing Prof. Semmelweis's Book on Puerperal Fever," *Medical Weekly* (1861): 13, cited in Gortvay and Zoltan, *Semmelweis*, 72.
3. Lesky, *Vienna Medical*, 186.
4. Gortvay and Zoltan, *Semmelweis*, 72.
5. Sillo-Seidl, *Wahrheit*, 12.
6. Lois Magner, *A History of Medicine* (New York: Marcel Dekker, 1992), 266.
7. Gortvay and Zoltan, *Semmelweis*, 72–73.
8. Gortvay and Zoltan, *Semmelweis*, 71.
9. Sinclair, *Semmelweis*, 148–49.
10. Sinclair, *Semmelweis*, 89.
11. Sinclair, *Semmelweis*, 119.
12. Gortvay and Zoltan, *Semmelweis*, 83–84.
13. Gortvay and Zoltan, *Semmelweis*, 84.
14. Sinclair, *Semmelweis*, 132.
15. Sinclair, *Semmelweis*, 119–20.
16. Irving I. Edgar, "Ignaz Phillip Semmelweis: Outline for a Biography," *Annals of Medical History* 1 (1939): 86.
17. Gortvay and Zoltan, *Semmelweis*, 85.

18. Semmelweis, *Etiology*, 413.
19. Gortvay and Zoltan, *Semmelweis*, 85–86.
20. Edgar, "Ignaz Phillip," 86–87.
21. Gortvay and Zoltan, *Semmelweis*, 86–88.
22. Gortvay and Zoltan, *Semmelweis*, 91.
23. Semmelweis, *Etiology*, 416.
24. Gortvay and Zoltan, *Semmelweis*, 94.
25. Edgar, "Ignaz Phillip," 88.
26. Semmelweis, *Etiology*, 416–17.
27. Nuland, *Doctors' Plague*, 146.
28. Edgar, "Ignaz Phillip," 89.
29. Edgar, "Ignaz Phillip," 90.
30. Edgar, "Ignaz Phillip," 91.
31. Edgar, "Ignaz Phillip," 94.
32. Gortvay and Zoltan, *Semmelweis*, 98–99.
33. Sinclair, *Semmelweis*, 132.
34. Gortvay and Zoltan, *Semmelweis*, 100.
35. Gortvay and Zoltan, *Semmelweis*, 89.
36. Gortvay and Zoltan, *Semmelweis*, 160.
37. Gortvay and Zoltan, *Semmelweis*, 160.
38. Sinclair, *Semmelweis*, 148.
39. Sinclair, *Semmelweis*, 150.
40. Sinclair, *Semmelweis*, 107.
41. Sinclair, *Semmelweis*, 152–53.
42. Gortvay and Zoltan, *Semmelweis*, 161.
43. Semmelweis, *Etiology*, 692–93.
44. Sinclair, *Semmelweis*, 144.
45. Semmelweis, *Etiology*, 762.
46. Sinclair, *Semmelweis*, 155.
47. Gortvay and Zoltan, *Semmelweis*, 162.
48. Sinclair, *Semmelweis*, 172.
49. Gortvay and Zoltan, *Semmelweis*, 163.
50. Sinclair, *Semmelweis*, 179–80.
51. Sinclair, *Semmelweis*, 181.
52. Sinclair, *Semmelweis*, 182–84.
53. Sinclair, *Semmelweis*, 182–83.
54. Sinclair, *Semmelweis*, 185–86.
55. Gortvay and Zoltan, *Semmelweis*, 145–46.
56. Sinclair, *Semmelweis*, 193–94.
57. Gortvay and Zoltan, *Semmelweis*, 107–08.

Aetiology

1. Gortvay and Zoltan, *Semmelweis*, 131.
2. Loudon, *Tragedy*, 103.
3. Loudon, *Tragedy*, 103.
4. Sinclair, *Semmelweis*, 197–98.
5. Sinclair, *Semmelweis*, 198.

6. Semmelweis, *Etiology*, 351–52.

7. Edgar, "Ignaz Phillip," 95.

8. Gortvay and Zoltan, *Semmelweis*, 134–35.

9. Sinclair, *Semmelweis*, 201.

10. Semmelweis, *Etiology*, 778.

11. Sinclair, *Semmelweis*, 201.

12. Sillo-Seidl, *Wahrheit*, 172.

13. Frederick K. Goodwin and Kay Redfield Jamison, *Manic-Depressive Illness: Bipolar Disorders and Recurrent Depression*, 2nd ed. (Oxford: Oxford University Press, 2007), 5–7.

14. Goodwin and Jamison, *Manic-Depressive*, 7–8.

15. David J. Miklowitz, *Bipolar Disorder: A Family-Focused Treatment Approach*, 2nd ed. (New York: The Guilford Press, 2008), 23.

16. Miklowitz, *Bipolar*, 61.

17. Sinclair, *Semmelweis*, 195.

18. Sinclair, *Semmelweis*, 202.

19. Sinclair, *Semmelweis*, 204.

20. Sinclair, *Semmelweis*, 205.

21. Sinclair, *Semmelweis*, 217.

22. Sinclair, *Semmelweis*, 209–10.

23. Sinclair, *Semmelweis*, 211–17.

24. Sinclair, *Semmelweis*, 223.

25. Sinclair, *Semmelweis*, 226.

26. Sinclair, *Semmelweis*, 227–28.

27. Semmelweis, *Etiology*, trans. Carter, 193.

28. Semmelweis, *Etiology*, trans. Carter, 194.

29. Semmelweis, *Etiology*, trans. Carter, 198.

30. Semmelweis, *Etiology*, trans. Carter, 202.

31. Semmelweis, *Etiology*, trans. Carter, 204, 364–65.

32. W. Friedrich Scanzoni, *Lehrbuch der Geburtschilfe*, 3rd ed. (Vienna: L. W. Seidl, 1855), 1, cited in Semmelweis, *Etiology*, trans. Carter, 208.

33. Scanzoni, *Lehrbuch*, 1,010, cited in Semmelweis, *Etiology*, trans. Carter, 208–9.

34. Scanzoni, *Lehrbuch*, 1,010, cited in Semmelweis, *Etiology*, trans. Carter, 209.

35. Loudon, *Tragedy*, 102.

36. Semmelweis, *Etiology*, trans. Carter, 211.

37. Semmelweis, *Etiology*, 669.

38. Semmelweis, *Etiology*, 670.

39. Semmelweis, *Etiology*, 668–71.

40. Semmelweis, *Etiology*, 671.

41. E. B. Krumbhaar, "The Centenary of the Cell Doctrine," *Annals of Medical History* 1 (1939): 436.

42. Semmelweis, *Etiology*, 714.

43. Semmelweis, *Etiology*, 713–14.

44. Semmelweis, *Etiology*, 723–24.

45. Semmelweis, *Etiology*, 729.

46. Semmelweis, *Etiology*, 730.

47. Ibid.
48. Semmelweis, *Etiology*, 731.
49. Semmelweis, *Etiology*, 732.
50. Semmelweis, *Etiology*, 733.
51. Semmelweis, *Etiology*, 738.
52. Semmelweis, *Etiology*, 737.
53. Semmelweis, *Etiology*, 738–45.
54. Semmelweis, *Etiology*, 771.
55. Ibid.
56. Ibid.
57. Semmelweis, *Etiology*, 762.
58. Semmelweis, *Etiology*, 762–63.
59. Semmelweis, *Etiology*, 772.

Reaction to *Aetiology*

1. Gortvay and Zoltan, *Semmelweis*, 140.
2. Sinclair, *Semmelweis*, 230–31.
3. Gortvay and Zoltan, *Semmelweis*, 140.
4. Ibid.
5. Gortvay and Zoltan, *Semmelweis*, 141.
6. Gortvay and Zoltan, *Semmelweis*, 138.
7. Sinclair, *Semmelweis*, 232.
8. Ibid.
9. Gortvay and Zoltan, *Semmelweis*, 141–43.
10. Sinclair, *Semmelweis*, 240–41.
11. Sinclair, *Semmelweis*, 236–37.
12. Sinclair, *Semmelweis*, 237–38.
13. Semmelweis, *Etiology*, xxxviii.
14. Gortvay and Zoltan, *Semmelweis*, 144.

Open Letters

1. Gortvay and Zoltan, *Semmelweis*, 144.
2. Gortvay and Zoltan, *Semmelweis*, 185.
3. Gortvay and Zoltan, *Semmelweis*, 144.
4. Gortvay and Zoltan, *Semmelweis*, 183.
5. Loudon, *Tragedy*, 104.
6. Istvan Benedek, "Betegsege es Halala," *Orvosi Hetilap*, 1971, April 18:112 (16) 930.
7. Benedek, "Betegsege," 929.
8. Gortvay and Zoltan, *Semmelweis*, 184.
9. Gortvay and Zoltan, *Semmelweis*, 183.
10. Gortvay and Zoltan, *Semmelweis*, 186.
11. Gortvay and Zoltan, *Semmelweis*, 182.
12. Semmelweis, *Etiology*, 784.
13. Semmelweis, *Etiology*, 785–86.
14. Semmelweis, *Etiology*, 786.

15. Gortvay and Zoltan, *Semmelweis*, 145.

16. Semmelweis, *Etiology*, 787.

17. Semmelweis, *Etiology*, 791.

18. Gortvay and Zoltan, *Semmelweis*, 146.

19. Semmelweis, *Etiology*, 794.

20. Sinclair, *Semmelweis*, 256.

21. Semmelweis, *Etiology*, 891.

22. Sinclair, *Semmelweis*, 252.

23. Sinclair, *Semmelweis*, 252.

24. Gortvay and Zoltan, *Semmelweis*, 149.

25. Sinclair, *Semmelweis*, 253.

26. Gortvay and Zoltan, *Semmelweis*, 149.

27. Gortvay and Zoltan, *Semmelweis*, 150.

28. Sinclair, *Semmelweis*, 241.

29. Gortvay and Zoltan, *Semmelweis*, 150.

30. Gortvay and Zoltan, *Semmelweis*, 152.

31. Gortvay and Zoltan, *Semmelweis*, 150.

32. Semmelweis, *Etiology*, 846–47.

33. Semmelweis, *Etiology*, 856–57.

34. Semmelweis, *Etiology*, 847.

35. Ibid.

36. Semmelweis, *Etiology*, 880.

37. Ibid.

38. Sinclair, *Semmelweis*, 257.

39. Semmelweis, *Etiology*, 777.

40. Gortvay and Zoltan, *Semmelweis*, 187.

41. Gortvay and Zoltan, *Semmelweis*, 186.

42. Gortvay and Zoltan, *Semmelweis*, 109–10.

43. Gortvay and Zoltan, *Semmelweis*, 110–13.

44. Theodore Duka, "Childbed Fever; Its Causes and Prevention: A Life's History," *Lancet* 2 (1886): 248.

45. Loudon, *Tragedy*, 104.

Illness and Descent

1. Loudon, *Tragedy*, 103.

2. Gortvay and Zoltan, *Semmelweis*, 184–86.

3. Loudon, *Tragedy*, 105.

4. Sillo-Seidl, *Wahrheit*, 150.

5. Kay Redfield Jamison, *An Unquiet Mind: A Memoir of Moods and Madness* (New York: Alfred A. Knopf, 2007), 218.

6. Hagop Akiskal, "Heterogeneity of Mood Disorders," in *Kaplan's and Sadock's Comprehensive Textbook of Psychiatry*, 9th ed., Vol. I (Philadelphia: Lippincott, 2009), 695–96.

7. Sinclair, *Semmelweis*, 267.

8. K. Codell Carter, Scott Abbott, and James L. Siebach, "Five Documents Relating to the Final Illness and Death of Ignaz Semmelweis," *Bulletin of the History of Medicine* 69 (1995): 258.

9. Duka, "Childbed Fever," 248.

10. Carter et al., "Five Documents," 261.

11. Sillo-Seidl, *Wahrheit*, 13.

12. Sillo-Seidl, *Wahrheit*, 170.

13. Sillo-Seidl, *Wahrheit*, 172.

14. Sillo-Seidl, *Wahrheit*, 169.

15. Carter et al., "Five Documents," 259–60.

16. Sillo-Seidl, *Wahrheit*, 172.

17. Carter et al., "Five Documents," 256.

18. Sillo-Seidl, *Wahrheit*, 207.

19. Sillo-Seidl, *Wahrheit*, 179.

20. Carter et al., "Five Documents," 260–61.

21. Sillo-Seidl, *Wahrheit*, 177–79.

22. Sillo-Seidl, *Wahrheit*, 177.

23. Loudon, *Tragedy*, 105.

24. Sillo-Seidl, *Wahrheit*, 13.

25. Carter et al., "Five Documents," 262.

26. Sillo-Seidl, *Wahrheit*, 14.

27. Sillo-Seidl, *Wahrheit*, 124.

28. Sillo-Seidl, *Wahrheit*, 177.

29. Sillo-Seidl, *Wahrheit*, 14.

30. Sillo-Seidl, *Wahrheit*, 152.

Lower Austrian Mental Asylum

1. Sillo-Seidl, *Wahrheit*, 145.

2. Sillo-Seidl, *Wahrheit*, 197.

3. Carter et al., "Five Documents," 265.

4. Gortvay and Zoltan, *Semmelweis*, 189.

5. Sillo-Seidl, *Wahrheit*, 181.

6. Sillo-Seidl, *Wahrheit*, 145.

7. Carter et al., "Five Documents," 263.

8. Sillo-Seidl, *Wahrheit*, 185–86.

9. Carter et al., "Five Documents," 264.

10. Sillo-Seidl, *Wahrheit*, 186.

11. Carter et al., "Five Documents," 264.

12. Carter et al., "Five Documents," 259–66.

13. Carter et al., "Five Documents," 268.

14. Benedek, "Betegsege," 113.

15. Semmelweis, *Etiology*, trans. Carter, 58.

16. Gortvay and Zoltan, *Semmelweis*, 192.

17. Carter et al., "Five Documents," 269.

18. Ibid.

19. Markusovsky, "Reviewing,"551–52, cited in Gortvay and Zoltan, *Semmelweis*, 194–95.

20. Carter et al., "Five Documents," 270.

21. Sinclair, *Semmelweis*, 270.

22. Gortvay and Zoltan, *Semmelweis*, 184.

23. Ibid.

24. G. Theodore Gram, "A Biographical Sketch of I. Ph. Semmelweis Commemorating the Antiseptic Method," (Philadelphia: 1898), cited in Gortvay and Zoltan, *Semmelweis*, 184.

25. Istvan Benedek, *Semmelweis and His Age* (Budapest: 1967), 415, cited in Gortvay and Zoltan, *Semmelweis*, 198.

26. William Hunter, "Chronic Sepsis as a Cause of Mental Disorder," *British Journal of Medicine* 5 (1927): 811–12.

27. P. O. Hasselgren and J. E. Fischer, "Septic Encephalopathy," *Intensive Care Medicine* 12 (1986): 13–16.

28. Hunter, "Chronic Sepsis," 815–18.

29. Miklowitz, *Bipolar*, 61.

30. Kay Redfield Jamison, *Touched with Fire: Manic-Depressive Illness and the Artistic Temperament* (New York: Free Press Paperbacks, 1993), 144–46.

31. Goodwin and Jamison, *Manic-Depressive*, 612–13 and plate 4.

32. E. J. Nestler, M. Barrot, R. J. DiLeone, et al., "Neurobiology of Depression," *Neuron* 34 (2002): 18–20.

33. Goodwin and Jamison, *Manic-Depressive*, plate 1, opposite 614.

Resurrection

1. Gortvay and Zoltan, *Semmelweis*, 171.

2. Gortvay and Zoltan, *Semmelweis*, 236.

3. Sinclair, *Semmelweis*, 262.

4. Josef Spaeth, "Statistische und historische Ruckblicke auf die Vorkommnisse des Wiener Gebarhauses wahrend die letzten 30 Jahre, mit besonderer Berucksichtigung der puerperalen Erkrankungen," *Med. Jahrbericht* 20 (1864): 145–64, cited in Loudon, *Tragedy*, 145–46.

5. Sinclair, *Semmelweis*, 290.

6. Sinclair, *Semmelweis*, 291.

7. Sinclair, *Semmelweis*, 60–61.

8. Sinclair, *Semmelweis*, 300–301.

9. Sinclair, *Semmelweis*, 301.

10. Sinclair, *Semmelweis*, 309.

11. Obenchain, *Victorian Vivisection*, 113.

12. Loudon, *Tragedy*, 121.

13. Loudon, *Tragedy*, 136.

14. Loudon, *Tragedy*, 137.

15. Loudon, *Tragedy*, 136–37.

16. Loudon, *Tragedy*, 142.

17. Duka, "Childbed Fever," 248.

18. Loudon, *Tragedy*, 148.

19. Gortvay and Zoltan, *Semmelweis*, 238.

20. Loudon, *Tragedy*, 148.

21. O. Pertik, "In Memoriam Semmelweis," Memorial Speech, Budapest, 1911, 15, cited in Gortvay and Zoltan, *Semmelweis*, 185.

22. Gortvay and Zoltan, *Semmelweis*, 238.

23. Loudon, *Tragedy*, 148.

24. Nuland, *Doctors' Plague*, 175.

25. Nuland, *Doctors' Plague*, 171.

26. Ibid.

27. Nuland, *Doctors' Plague*, 174–75.

28. Nuland, *Doctors' Plague*, 171.

29. Nuland, *Doctors' Plague*, 172–73.

30. Carl Sagan, *The Demon-Haunted World: Science as a Candle in the Dark* (New York: Ballantine Books, 1997), 304.

31. Nuland, *Doctors' Plague*, 179.

32. Nuland, *Doctors' Plague*, 183.

33. Codell Carter, "Semmelweis and His Predecessors," *Medical History* 25 (1981): 72.

34. Slaughter, *Immortal Magyar*, 206.

35. Sinclair, *Semmelweis*, 368–69.

36. Semmelweis, *Etiology*, 772.

Bibliography

Akiskal, Hagop. "Heterogeneity of Mood Disorders." In *Kaplan's and Sadock's Comprehensive Textbook of Psychiatry*, 9th ed., Vol. 1, 1693–1706. Philadelphia: Lippincott (2009).

Alexander, Jessy J., Alexander Jakob, Patrick Cunningham, et al. "TNF is a Key Mediator of Septic Encephalopathy Acting through its Receptor, TNF Receptor-1." *Neurochemistry International* 52 (2008): 447–56.

Andreason, N. C. "Symptoms, Signs and Diagnosis of Schizophrenia." *Lancet* 347 (1995): 477–81.

Antall, Jozsef, ed. *Medical History in Hungary, 1972*. Budapest: Medicina Konyvkiado (1972).

Arneth, Franz Hektor. "Evidence of Puerperal Fever Depending on the Contagious Inoculation of Morbid Matter." *Monthly Journal of Medical Science* 12 (1851): 505–11.

Ashworth Underwood, E. *Boerhaave's Men: At Leyden and After*. Edinburgh: Edinburgh University Press (1977).

Balfour, George W. "English and German Midwives." *Lancet* 2 (1855): 503.

Benedek, Istvan. "Betegsege es Halala," *Orvosi Hetilap* (1971): 929–36.

———. *Semmelweis and His Age*. Budapest: Akamemiai Kiado (1967).

Bennett, Ezra P. "On the Identity of Erysipelas and a Certain Form of Puerperal Fever and its Contagiousness." *American Journal of Medical Sciences* 19 (1850): 376–83.

Boehr, Max. "Untersuchungen uber die Haufigkeit des Todes im Wochenbett in Preussen." *Zeitschrift fur Geburtschulfe und Gynekologie* 3 (1878): 17–151.

Boerhaave, Herman. *Aphorisms Concerning the Knowledge and Cure of Diseases*. Translated by J. Del Acoste. London: B. Cowsend and W. Innys, 1715. https://archive.org/details/boerhaavesaphor00delagoog.

Campbell, W. "On Puerperal Fever." *London Medical Gazette* 9 (1831–2): 353–54.

Carter, Codell. "Ignaz Semmelweis, Carl Mayhofer and the Rise of Germ Theory." *Medical History* 29 (1985): 33–53.

———. *Ignaz Semmelweis, The Etiology, Concept, and Prophylaxis of Childbed Fever*. Madison: The University of Wisconsin Press (1983).

―――. "Semmelweis and His Predecessors." *Medical History*, 25 (1981): 57–72.

Carter, K. Codell, and Barbara Carter. *Childbed Fever: A Scientific Biography of Ignaz Semmelweis*. Westport, CT: Greenwood Press (1994).

Carter, K. Codell, and George S. Tate. "The Earliest-Known Account of Semmelweis's Initiation of Disinfection at Vienna's Allegemeines Krankenhaus." *Bulletin of the History of Medicine* 65 (1991): 252–57.

―――. "Josef Skoda's Relationship to the work of Ignaz Semmelweis." *Medizin Historisches Journal* 19 (1984): 335–47.

Carter, K. Codell, Scott Abbott, and James L. Siebach. "Five Documents Relating to the Final Illness and Death of Ignaz Semmelweis." *Bulletin of the History of Medicine* 69 (1995): 255–70.

"Cassandra of Troy." www.britannica.com/EBchecked/topic/9808/cassandra.

Chartier, Christian, and Edouard Grosshans. "Erysipelas." *International Journal of Dermatology* 29 (1990): 459–67.

Conway, David A., and Ronald Munson. *The Elements of Reasoning*, 3rd ed. Belmont, CA: Wadsworth/Thompson Learning (2000).

Cooper, Sir Astley Paston. "Surgical Lectures." *Lancet* 1 (1823): 1–9.

Csendes, Peter. *Historical Dictionary of Vienna*. London: The Scarecrow Press, Inc. (1999).

Cullingworth, Charles J. "Oliver Wendell Holmes and the Contagiousness of Puerperal Fever." *Jnl. Obstetrics and Gynecology British Empire* 8 (1905): 369–92.

Davies, Norman. *Europe: A History*. Oxford: Oxford University Press, 1996.

Dawson, Percy M. "Semmelweis, An Interpretation." *Annals of Medical History* 6 (1924): 258–79.

Del Acoste, J. *Boerhaave's Aphorisms Concerning the Knowledge and Cure of Diseases*. London: B. Cowse and W. Innys (1715).

DeLacy, Margaret. "Puerperal Fever in Eighteenth Century Britain." *Bulletin of the History of Medicine* 63 (1989): 521–56.

Dewhurst, Kenneth. *Doctor Thomas Sydenham: 1624–1689*. Berkeley: University of California Press (1966).

―――. *Oxford Medicine: Essays on the Evolution of the Oxford Clinical School to Commemorate the Bicentenary of the Radcliffe Infirmary 1770–1970*. Oxford: Sandford Publications (1970).

Dormandy, Thomas. *Moments of Truth: Four Creators of Modern Medicine*. Chichester: John Wiley and Sons (2003).

Duka, Theodore. "Childbed Fever; Its Causes and Prevention: A Life's History." *Lancet* 2 (1886): 206–08.

Edgar, Irving I. "Ignaz Phillip Semmelweis: Outline for a Biography." *Annals of Medical History* 1 (1939): 74–96.

Farmer, Alan. *World and Its Peoples: Central Europe*, Vol. 7. New York: Marshall Cavendish Reference (2010).

Fry, R. M. "Fatal Infection by Hemolytic Streptococci Group B." *Lancet* 1 (1938): 199.

Garber, James J. *Harmony and Healing: The Theoretical Basis for Ancient and Medieval Medicine*. New Brunswick: Transaction Publishers (2008).

Goodwin, Frederick K., and Kay Redfield Jamison. *Manic-Depressive Ill-*

ness: Bipolar Disorders and Recurrent Depression, 2nd ed. Oxford: Oxford University Press (2007).

Gortvay, Gyorgy, and Imre Zoltan. *Semmelweis: His Life and Work*. Budapest, Hungary: Akademiai Kiado, 1968.

Gram, G. Theodore. "A Biographical Sketch of I. Ph. Semmelweis Commemorating the Antiseptic Method." Philadelphia (1898): 184.

Gyorgyey, Ferenc A. *Puerperal Fever 1847–1861: From the First Statement about the Discovery to the Publication of Semmelweis's Aetiology*. Master's thesis, Yale University (1968).

Hasselgren, P. O., and J. E. Fischer. "Septic Encephalopathy." *Intensive Care Medicine* 12 (1986): 13–16.

Hervieux, Jacques Francois Edouard. *Traité clinique et pratique des maladies puerperales suite de couches*. Translated by I. Loudon. Paris (1880).

Hippocrates. *Hippocrates on Airs, Waters, and Places*. Translated by Emile Litre, Janus Cornarius, Johannes Antonides van der Linden, and Francis Adams. London: Wyman and Sons (1881).

Holmes, Oliver W. "On the Contagiousness of Puerperal Fever." *The New England Quarterly Journal of Medicine* 1 (1842–43): 503–30.

Hudson Garrison, Fielding. *An Introduction to the History of Medicine*, 3rd ed. Philadelphia: W. B. Saunders, 1922. Hunter, William. "Chronic Sepsis as a Cause of Mental Disorder." *British Journal of Medicine* 5 (1927): 811–18.

Hunter, William. "Chronic Sepsis as a Cause of Mental Disorder," *British Journal of Medicine* 5 (1927): 811–12.

Jablensky, A. "The Diagnostic Concept of Schizophrenia: Its History, Evolution and Future Prospects." *Dialogues Clinical Neuroscience* 12 (2010): 271–87.

Jackson, Alan C., Joseph J. Gilbert, Bryan Young, et al. "The Encephalopathy of Sepsis." *Le Journal Canadien des Sciences Neurologiques* 12 (1985): 303–7.

Jacob, H. E. *Johann Straus, Father and Son: A Century of Light Music*. Translated by Marguerite Wolff. Vancouver: Greystone Press (1940).

Jamison, Kay Redfield. *Touched with Fire: Manic-Depressive Illness and the Artistic Temperament*. New York: Free Press Paperbacks (1993).

———. *An Unquiet Mind: A Memoir of Moods and Madness*. New York: Alfred A. Knopf (2007).

Jetter, Dieter. *Geschichte des Hospitals*, Vol. 1. Wiesbaden: F. Steiner (1966).

King, Lester S. "Some Problems of Causality in Eighteenth Century Medicine." *Bulletin of the History of Medicine* 37 (1963): 15–24.

———. *The Medical World of the Eighteenth Century*. Chicago: The University of Chicago Press (1958).

Korns, Horace M. "A Brief History of Physical Diagnosis." *Annals of Medical History* 1 (1939): 50–67.

Krumbhaar, E. B., "The Centenary of the Cell Doctrine." *Annals of Medical History* 1 (1939): 427–37.

Kucher, Joseph. *Puerperal Convalescence and the Diseases of the Puerperal Period*. New York: Vail, 1886.

Leake, John. *Practical Observations on the Child-bed Fever*. 1772; reprinted in *Essays on the Puerperal Fever*, edited by Gleetwood Churchill, London: Sydenham Society (1849).

Lesky, Erna. *The Vienna Medical School of the 19th Century*. Baltimore: The Johns Hopkins University Press (1976).

Lindeboom, G. A. *Herman Boerhaave: The Man and His Work*. London: Methuen & Co. (1968).

Lombard, F. H. "Puerperal Fever, Prophylaxis in Hospital Practice, Notes on the Lying-in Hospitals of Vienna, Dresden and Prague." *Boston Medical and Surgical Journal* 108 (1883): 509–11.

Loudon, Irvine. *Childbed Fever: A Documentary History*. New York: Garland Publishing (1995).

———. "Puerperal Fever, the Streptococcus and the Sulfonamides." *British Medical Journal* 295 (1987): 485–90.

———. *The Tragedy of Childbed Fever*. Oxford: Oxford University Press (2000).

Magner, Lois. *A History of Medicine*. New York: Marcel Dekker (1992).

Major, Ralph H. *A History of Medicine*, Vol. 2. Springfield: Charles C. Thomas (1954).

Meigs, Charles D. *Females and Their Diseases; A Series of Letters to His Class*. Philadelphia: Lea and Blanchard (1848).

Merriman, John. *A History of Modern Europe: From the Renaissance to the Present*. New York: W. W. Norton and Company (2010).

Merriman, John, and Jay Winter. *Europe 1789 to 1914: Encyclopedia of the Age of Industry and Empire*, Vol. 1. Detroit: Thompson Gale (2006).

Miklowitz, David J. *Bipolar Disorder: A Family-Focused Treatment Approach*, 2nd ed. New York: The Guilford Press (2008).

Miller, C. M. "On the Treatment of Puerperal Fever." *Lancet* 2 (1848): 262–71.

Murphy, Frank P. "Ignaz Philipp Semmelweis: An Annotated Bibliography." *Bulletin of the History of Medicine* 20 (1946): 653–70.

National Institutes of Health/National Library of Medicine. "Schizophrenia." *MedlinePlus*. Accessed March 15, 2012. http://www.nlm.nih.gov/medlineplus/ency/article/000928.htm.

Nestler, E. J., M. Barrot, R. J. DiLeone, et al. "Neurobiology of Depression." *Neuron* 34 (2002): 13–25.

Nuland, Sherwin B. *Doctors: The Biography of Medicine*. New York: Knopf (1988).

———. *The Doctors' Plague: Germs, Childbed Fever, and the Strange Story of Ignac Semmelweis*. New York: W. W. Norton Company (2003).

———. "The Enigma of Semmelweis—An Interpretation." *Journal of the History of Medicine and Allied Sciences* 34 (1979): 255–72.

Obenchain, Theodore G. *The Victorian Vivisection Debate: Frances Power Cobbe, Experimental Science and the "Claims of Brutes."* Jefferson, NC: McFarland and Company, Inc. (2012).

Papadopoulos, Marios, C. Ceri Davies, Ray Moss, et al. "Pathophysiology of Septic Encephalopathy: A Review." *Critical Care Medicine* 28 (2000): 3019–24.

Porter, Roy. *Blood and Guts: A Short History of Medicine*. London: W. W. Norton and Company (2002).

Robinson, Victor. "Pathfinders in Medicine: Semmelweis, the Obstetrician." *Medical Review of Reviews* 18 (1912): 232–46.

Rothstein, William G. *American Physicians in the Nineteenth Century: From Sects to Science*. Baltimore: The Johns Hopkins University Press (1985).

Routh, C. H. F. "On the Causes of the Endemic Puerperal Fever of Vienna." *Medico-Chirurgical Transactions* 32 (1849): 27–40.

Sagan, Carl. *The Demon-Haunted World: Science as a Candle in the Dark*. New York: Ballantine Books (1997).

Schurer von Waldheim, Fritz. *Ignaz Phillip Semmelweis, Sein Leben und Wirken. Urteile der Mit- und Nachwelt*. Wien and Leipzig: A. Hartleben (1904).

Seligman, Stanley. "The Lesser Pestilence: Non-epidemic Puerperal Fever." *Medical History* 35 (1991): 89–102.

Semmelweis, Ignaz. *The Etiology, the Concept and the Prophylaxis of Childbed Fever*. Translated by Frank P. Murphy. With *Open Letters*, translated by Sherwin B. Nuland and Ferenc A. Gyorgyey. The Classics of Surgery Library Special Edition. New York: Gryphon Editions (1994).

Shakespeare, William. *The Merchant of Venice*. Accessed November 19, 2015. http://www.opensourceshakespeare.org/.

Shorter, Edward. *A History of Women's Bodies*. London: Allen Lane (1983).

Sillo-Seidl, Georg. *Die Wahrheit uber Semmelweis: Eine Bild-Biographie*. Translated by Lori Schultheis. Genf: Ariston Verlag (1978).

Sinclair, H. M. "Some Ups and Downs of Oxford Science." In *Oxford Medicine: Essays on the Evolution of the Oxford Clinical School to Commemorate the Bicentenary of the Radcliffe Infirmary, 1770–1970*, edited by Kenneth Dewhurst, Oxford: Sandford Publications (1970).

Sinclair, William. *Semmelweis: His Life and His Doctrine*. Manchester: Manchester University Press (1909).

Skoda, Josef. *A Treatise on Percussion and Auscultation*, trans. W. O. Markham, 4th ed. London: Highly and Son (1853).

Slaughter, Frank G. *Immortal Magyar*. New York: Henry Schuman (1950).

Tandon, Rajiv, Matcheri S. Keshavon, and Henry A. Nasrallah. "Schizophrenia, 'Just the Facts' What We Know in 2008. 2. Epidemiology and Etiology." *Schizophrenia Research* 102 (2008): 1–18.

Tandon, Rajiv, Henry A. Nasrallah, and Matcheri S. Keshavon. "Schizophrenia, 'Just the Facts' 4. Clinical Features and Conceptualization." *Schizophrenia Research* 110 (2009): 1–23.

Thomas, Lewis. *The Fragile Species*. New York: Charles Scribner's Sons (1992).

———. *The Youngest Scientist; Notes of a Medical Watcher*. New York: Penguin Books (1983).

Thompson, John D., and Grace Goldin. *The Hospital: A Social and Architectural History*. New Haven: Yale University Press (1975).

Thompson, Morton. *The Cry and the Covenant*. New York: Doubleday (1949).

Tillmanns, Herman. *Textbook of Surgery*. New York: D. Appleton and Company (1901): 347.

Trail, R. R. "Sydenham's Impact on English Medicine." *Medical History* 9

(1965): 356–64. Accessed November 19, 2015. http://www.ncbi.nlm.nih.gov/pmc/articles/PMC1033532/.

Van Os, J., and S. Kapur. "Schizophrenia." *Lancet* 374 (2009): 635–45.

Virchow, Rudolf. "Uber die nosologische und Atiologische Stellung des Epidemischen Puerperalfiebers." *Monatschr. F. Gebertsk. U. Frauenkr* 23 (1864): 406–12.

Wangensteen, Owen H. "Nineteenth Century Wound Management of the Parturient Uterus and Compound Fracture: The Semmelweis–Lister Priority Controversy." *Bulletin of the New York Academy of Medicine* 46 (1970): 565–96.

Winckel, Franz von. "Ignaz Phillip Semmelweis." *Munchener medizinische Wochenschrift* 40 (1893): 871–74.

Yost, R. M. "Sydenham's Philosophy of Science." *Osiris* 9 (1950): 84–105. Accessed May 29, 2009. http://www.jstor.org/stable/301845.

Young, Ignatius J. "The Respective Merits of Semmelweis and Oliver Wendell Holmes in the Treatment of Childbed Fever." *Lancet* 1 (1907): 179.

Index